Books by Lorus *and* Margery Milne

THE SENSES OF ANIMALS AND MEN 1962

THE MOUNTAINS 1962

THE BALANCE OF NATURE 1960

THE LOWER ANIMALS
LIVING INVERTEBRATES OF THE WORLD 1960
WITH RALPH AND MILDRED BUCHSBAUM

ANIMAL LIFE 1959

PLANT LIFE 1959

PATHS ACROSS THE EARTH 1958

THE WORLD OF NIGHT 1956

THE MATING INSTINCT 1954

THE BIOTIC WORLD AND MAN 1952, 1958

FAMOUS NATURALISTS 1952

A MULTITUDE OF LIVING THINGS 1947

THE
SENSES
OF
ANIMALS
AND
MEN

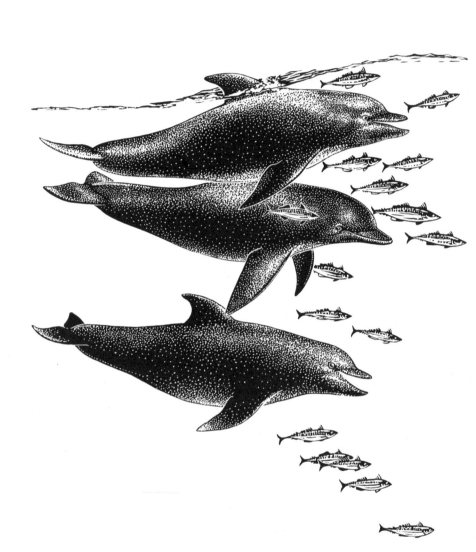

Lorus *and* Margery Milne

THE
SENSES
OF
ANIMALS
AND
MEN

Drawings by Kenneth Gosner

ATHENEUM : NEW YORK

1962

We wish to express our appreciation to the Curtis Publishing Company of Philadelphia for permission to quote from Dame Edith Sitwell's "Adventure of the Mind" in the November 15, 1958, issue of the *Saturday Evening Post;* to Doubleday & Company, Inc., Garden City, New York, for the quotation from the late Roy Bedichek's *The Sense of Smell* (1960); to Yale University Press, New Haven, Connecticut, for permission to quote Dr. Donald R. Griffin from *Listening in the Dark* (1958); to *American Scholar*, *Atlantic Monthly*, and *Scientific American* for allowing us to quote freely from our own articles entitled respectively "What Do Animals See?" (Winter, 1958-59), "How Cool Is a Cucumber?" (April, 1948), and "Insect Vision" (July, 1948).

TO *Claude* AND *Jean*
AND THE EXCITING
SENSE OF DISCOVERY
IN LA JOLLA

A Sense of Wonder

IN CITY and country, on land and ship and plane, people have asked us a reasonable question: "What led you to devote your lives to the study of living things?" We have never needed to ask ourselves.

Other fields, admittedly, have fascinated us; we have digressed enough to know what immense satisfactions are waiting elsewhere. But from each delightful digression we find ourselves returning as though coming home to the diversity of modern animals and plants, to the stupendous history that has led to them and us, and to the dynamic web that links together these wonderful living things. Where else, we ask ourselves, could we find anything so challenging, so intricately organized and, at the same time, so capable of fluid change? Each new discovery emphasizes this sense of wonder.

We suspect that the scientist and the poet have more in common than either of them ordinarily admits. The sense of wonder reaches both. We believe it was the sense Dame Edith Sitwell had in mind when she wrote of any good poet that "Like Moses, he sees God in the burning bush when the half-opened or myopic physical eye sees only the gardener burning leaves." The sense of wonder seems to slip over a special part of a person's self, and to fit so well that the world thereafter seems different, more pleasing, more important. The lure of the unknown grows clearer, even irresistible.

Is the capacity to wonder and admire not one of the few characteristics really distinguishing man from nonhuman life? New discoveries of science need not distract our attention until we notice only the colossal in size, in cost, in power, in physical overdevelopment. They can serve instead to increase the sense of wonder we had as a child, by opening the mind to vistas of which we had not dreamed. At the same time we can cherish our sense of wonder over things science makes no real attempt to explain: the symmetry in a daisy or an orchid, the texture of petals or fur, the fragrance of a wild rose or a yarrow leaf, the darting flash of a dragonfly or a hummingbird, the twinkling messages of fireflies in the dusk, the cheer in the call of a chickadee, or the social organization in a beehive.

As we think about the animal kingdom, its ultimate wonder seems to lie in the adaptive awarenesses that link each individual with its neighbors, that may be developed into deliberate communication, and that make civilization possible. The sensory perception shown by animals is their most distinctive trait, separating them from the plants. Awareness seems far more significant than movements, for without senses the motility would be largely meaningless.

But what should be counted as a sense? Is it merely those combinations of living matter and a coordinating mechanism, whether within a single cell or at distinctive sites within a multicellular animal? Vision means more to a firefly than just seeing in daylight. By producing light as well as detecting it, these insects can communicate visually at night when otherwise they would be blind. To a honeybee, vibrations mean more than just variations in pressure or any simple extension of touch. These senses have become part of an elaborate counterpart of language. By expending energy, animals are able to broaden their awarenesses, to extend their basic senses. So can we.

For years now, we have enjoyed little demonstrations of awareness among animals and men, alert sensitivities to the living environment that prove how broad is the spectrum of sensation. Our thanks go to Hiram Haydn, who invited us to spread these pleasures of ours on the pages of *American Scholar*, and then followed with warm letters urging us to weave a fuller story into the form of the present book. In writing the chapters we have relived many of our own experiences with animals on four continents. We would like to share and make contagious our own special sense of wonder.

L.J.M. and M.M.

Durham, New Hampshire

Contents

THE
SENSES
OF
ANIMALS
AND
MEN

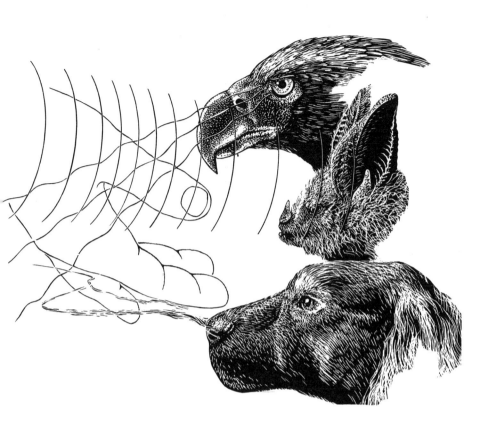

1. *The "Five Senses" and a Few More*

THE WORLD is known to us through many senses, not just hearing, smell, vision and, at close range, touch and taste. Aristotle recognized these five, setting a pattern that has been followed for more than two thousand years. Like men before him, Aristotle was impressed by small numbers. Five senses fitted into a magic series: one True Cause, two Sexes, three Graces, four Humors. Today the chain continues. Every Irishman can name the Six Counties. We refer to the seven wonders of the world, the eight notes in an octave, the cat's nine lives. Such numbers are handy, even if oversimplified.

Touch seems simple too. It tells us of the presence and

3

shape of a stone in the dark, but not that it is cool. Our skins contain special endings from the nervous system, keeping the brain aware whether our bodies are gaining heat or losing it. We lose heat to a stone in the dark. Unless, of course, our fingers have been in a container of ice water. Then the stone may be warmer than our fingers, and from it heat will flow into the skin, telling us that the stone we touch is "warm." It is disconcerting to the brain if the skin of one warm hand reports that a certain stone is cool to the touch, at the same moment that the skin of the other —the chilled one—reports that the identical stone is warm. Which hand should we believe?

Our skins let us know whether the air is humid or dry, whether surfaces are wet without being sticky or slippery. From the uniformity of slight pressure, we can be aware how deeply a finger is thrust into water at body temperature, even if the finger is encased in a rubber glove that keeps the skin completely dry. Many other animals, with highly sensitive skins, appear able to learn still more about their environment. Often they do so without employing any of the five senses Aristotle knew.

The first sense to be measured quantitatively was none of the famous five. A century ago Ernst Weber tested his own ability, and then that of others, to tell which was the heavier of two weights held one in each hand. He discovered that this sensitivity is relative and not absolute.

Most people can judge that an object weighing 82 grams (2.89 ounces) is heavier than one weighing 80 grams (2.82 ounces), or that 4.1 pounds is more than 4.0 pounds, or 41 pounds more than 40. Any lesser difference is beyond the limits of our sense of weight. For all senses tested since Weber's time, the "just discriminable difference" has this ratio form. Differences of two per cent are about as fine as the nervous system will appreciate. This is a measure of our sense of contrast.

Sometimes we describe ourselves as being "a bit under the weather," without realizing that this may be true. In Europe recently, factory workers were found to show slower mental activity, more mistakes and a higher accident rate when the barometer was falling and a storm on its way, than under a rising barometer and clearing skies.

So far no one has discovered where the sensitivity to weather resides in the body. The man who claimed he could predict rain because his amputated leg ached before the clouds gathered may have been telling the truth. In the inner ear, our organs of balance have no role in hearing, no connection to smell, vision, touch or taste. Yet, if they are stimulated in unfamiliar patterns by movements of the body as a whole, they can give rise to air sickness, sea sickness and car sickness, miseries that are aggravated by what we see and smell. The most experienced and determined man is unable to tolerate prolonged stimulation of these organs of balance. No person is immune to motion sickness if his intact inner-ear mechanisms are kept in a state of agitation. For this reason, would-be astronauts are practicing daily, learning to control their positions in weight-free space.

Some people and many animals seem to have a sense of direction, one independent of the familiar modes of awareness. Women sometimes accept this as an ordinary part of their extraordinary "feminine intuition." Perhaps everyone has capabilities in this way. But most of us are baffled in any attempt to draw on an unconscious store of compass information. Comparatively few of us can control the muscles that could wiggle our ears either, although this implies no absence of muscles or of nerve connections to them. It is only when an animal is unable to use the ordinary cues in finding its way about that its brain reaches for vaguer senses which are better than none at all.

Long ago, scientists discovered an easy way to demonstrate a vague sensitivity of this kind in ordinary frogs. When a healthy frog is placed in an observation box, about two feet in each direction, and light is admitted from only one side, the frog will turn to face the window and perhaps hop toward the light. If that window is covered and one on the opposite side opened, the frog turns around and again may hop toward the source of radiant energy. "Of course," we say. "It sees the light. After all, it has good eyes."

To respond in this way the frog actually needs neither its eyes nor most of its brain. Anyone can manage the simple surgery required to remove these organs. Unlike man, the frog will survive for weeks although unable to feed or to breathe except through its moist skin. When such a frog is placed in the test box with light admitted through only one side, the animal will turn and face the open window — even though a pane of glass prevents any current of air from entering with the light. The frog may hop or creep toward the stimulus. If that window is covered and one on the opposite side is opened, the frog detects the change and turns around. Its whole skin is sensitive to light. How much can a blind man use his skin in a comparable way? The feat might be just as possible as learning to wiggle the ears, and a great deal more useful.

Today the zoologist and the engineer are working together as never before, exploring the animal kingdom for ideas that might be applied to human needs. In a way, they are climbing down a few rungs on the evolutionary ladder, seeking to benefit from the accumulated experience of all other kinds of animate life. Actually, all creatures have an ancestry of approximately the same total length as man's own. For perhaps a billion years these many lines of descent have been diverging. Natural selection has been constantly channeling the inherited variability of each species into the form of adaptations. With these the many ancestral types escaped extinction, despite changes in their environment. The accumulated adaptations recognizable today mirror the long history of successful experiences along each separate line of descent.

These new endeavors are beginning to answer another question, one over which people have vacillated for years. Do animals have senses we lack, or do animal senses differ from ours merely in the degree of development they show? If there are indeed senses we lack but animals possess, we should be able to expand man's sensory world in those directions too, through workable imitations. All gains from these devices would supplement what has already been accomplished in extending our own major outward senses, and yield still broader avenues for messages to the human brain.

We are so conscious of our five famous senses that it is easy to overlook other ways in which the brain gets information. Our brain and spinal cord are remarkably efficient. Together they monitor innumerable sense organs affected by processes inside the body, and attend to almost every one of these without disturbing our consciousness. Sense organs in the brain itself respond to slight changes in the temperature of the blood, giving us a thermostat that keeps our blood temperature constant. In coded messages these centers advise the central nervous system, bringing about automatic adjustment in the rates of heat production and of heat loss. Other centers in the brain keep track of the carbon-dioxide content of the blood, and serve in regulating our breathing movements. Sensory endings in the wall of the alimentary canal, in the heart and blood vessels, serve unconscious mechanisms controlling the movement of food undergoing digestion and of blood carrying its astonishing load of foods, wastes, hormones, respiratory gases and agents protecting us from disease.

That we are so conscious of five senses is itself remarkable. The vast majority of animals rely upon almost completely automatic responses known as reflexes and instincts. These depend, in turn, upon nervous pathways linking muscles and glands to eyes and ears, organs of taste and of smell, and body surfaces sensitive to touch. Let a tabby cat merely hear a dog barking, even on a phonograph record, and she reacts. If no dog is visible, the cat may show no movements. Yet the soles of her feet begin to perspire. They get wet enough to complete an electrical circuit if she is standing on an ingenious piece of psychological test equipment—and a bell rings! The bell means nothing to the cat, but it proves to the experimenter that she has an automatic response to the sound of the unseen dog.

Scratch a dog's side and the animal's rear foot comes up to do the scratching. Rub the side of a parrot's head back where the lower jaw is hinged and the bird yawns compulsively. Have a person be the first living creature a duckling sees upon hatching, and thereafter the little bird is permanently "imprinted" by mankind—clearly convinced that it is no duckling but another human being.

One of our pet parakeets (budgerigars) is utterly unresponsive to the other budgies. She won't fly with them or stay if they come too close. But she'll rub noses with any human friend, will puff out her face feathers like green jowls and constrict her pupils in excitement. She's far more interested in licking milk from a cereal spoon than in pecking bird seed. And we can't eat an apple in her presence without giving her a slice   unless we want to see her do acrobatics in her cage and hear a whole repertory of attention-calling chatter. If we let her have her way, she'd perch on our shoulders all day!

Some of our own reactions are unnecessary. How often do we brace ourselves to keep from ducking as the delicate branch tips of a low limb are about to strike the sturdy windshield of our automobile passing under a tree? We can prevent ourselves from ducking, but not from blinking at the moment of contact. Or at the clinic, we sit on a table with our legs hung over the edge and see that the physician is about to tap us lightly on the kneecap with a rubber hammer. Our lower leg still kicks out. We know the tap is coming, and the reflex makes no sense except to the physician. Our nervous system provides the pathways and the stimulus leads to a prompt response.

With outward movements we respond also to the inner calls of hunger and hormones. Just as a caged rat will enter the exercise drum and run more often as its hunger increases, so will a lecture audience unconsciously shuffle feet and squirm more often in the seats as mealtime approaches.

All animals are surrounded ordinarily by a sea of stimuli to which they are sensitive. Yet most creatures react only to those stimuli related directly to sensations originating simultaneously within the body. Hunger, thirst, sexual readiness or some other internal drive may induce the animal to move about. This movement leads to nothing meaningful unless some external stimulus gives it direction. The texture of a leaf invites a hungry wanderer to bite and eat, or the sight of a shining pond, a glistening dew drop or a potential mate triggers some definite action serving to release the inner drive, to direct it and bring a reward.

Too seldom do we have the patience to watch the courtship antics of a bird or insect to their conclusion. We give up while the enthusiastic male continues working hard at his display because the mate he woos ignores him, continuing to preen or eat. His antics mean nothing to her until her reproductive system reaches the correct stage. Then and not before will his courtship signals serve their purpose. The male's elaborate gestures may elicit no outward movement on her part to show that she has noticed. Yet her nervous system may have responded, inducing her glands to pour hormones into her blood, indirectly speeding the development of her eggs. The hen pigeon will lay only if she hears the cooings of her mate. The adult female rat becomes sexually receptive soon after she is placed in a cage whose floor and walls offer her the exciting odor of adult male rats that have occupied it previously.

When any potential mother's eggs are ready, her brain receives new stimuli from her reproductive organs. Unless this happens, she is unlikely to respond to the male. She may actually repel him, as though he irritated her by his persistent attentions. Out of this paradoxical behavior comes our description of the female as the "contrary" sex!

The time of year serves also as a stimulus to which no sudden outward response can be expected. Spring, we say, is the season when "the young man's fancy lightly turns" more compulsively toward the opposite sex. Nutritionists have linked the change and the frequency of June marriages to vitamin deficiencies developed during winter months when fresh fruits and vegetables are scarcer than in summer and at harvest time. But now their explanation has become suspect. Certainly it will not account for the differences in a pasture where Dorset sheep and Shropshire sheep graze side by side. Dorsets choose spring as mating time, and lose their amatory interests when the weather turns summery. Shropshires mate in the fall, when deer and elk and moose are readying for the rut. Shepherds depend upon this difference in timing to prevent hybridization when the two breeds of sheep are pastured together, eating the same foods.

Whenever the summer proves to be unusually cool and cloudy, the Dorset sheep show no awareness that spring is over. On the other hand, the Shropshires are deceived by early dusks each day, by dark mornings and cool nights. They begin mating prematurely, acting in July as though it were September. Hybrids appear in this way, with both breeds lambing in winter and upsetting the shepherds' market calculations.

Dorsets react by readying themselves for reproduction when the days are long, the nights short in spring. Shropshires respond to the other proportions — shortening days and lengthening nights — during cool autumn weather. In normal years, sheep are so clearly regulated that this can be regarded as no mere "fancy." The ratio of night to day can account for the human response to springtime as well — far more convincingly today than any nutritional changes. We have no reason to regard ourselves as immune to the gradual alterations in night length, so characteristic of the outdoor year in temperate latitudes.

By observing the capabilities of other members of the animal kingdom, we come to realize that a human being has far more possibilities than are utilized. We neglect ever so many of our senses in concentrating on the five most conspicuous ones. At the same time, a comparison between animals and man draws attention to the limitations of each sense. The part of the spectrum seen by color-conscious man as red is nonexistent for owls and honeybees. But a bee or a butterfly can see far more in many flowers than we, because the ultraviolet to which our eyes are blind is a stimulating part of the insect's spectrum and, for honeybees at least, constitutes a separate color.

Differences in the importance of various senses to the many kinds of animals must alter their understanding of the world about them. The dog's world is one full of intriguing odors, the bat's a place of meaningful echoes, the hawk's a mosaic of finely seen details among which some features of movement betray a mouse or a grasshopper for dinner. Until we recognize these differences, it is almost impossible for us to understand our animal neighbors.

Not all of our senses are equally helpful to us. Despite the real comfort gained from the touch of a loved one or the delights we find in odors and flavors, we seldom rely upon these avenues of contact and chemical awareness. Just two senses stand out, as is evident in the renowned trio of little ivory monkeys on the shrine at Nikko, which are unconcerned about touch or taste or evil smells. Their admonitory poses relate instead to sound and light, which stimulate the senses we find most valuable in communication, navigation and detection of things at a distance. To some extent we can educate our senses by alerting the brain, for the messages it receives from our many sense organs do not themselves bring understanding. It is only when the brain compares an incoming pattern of sensory stimulation with past experience, either personal or vicarious, that something meaningful can emerge. This is the way we can sharpen our perception and increase our enjoyment of life.

Experience does nothing, however, to broaden the physical limits of our awareness. Always our sense organs remain the narrow windows through which our brain views the world. To reach beyond they must be supplemented with scientific devices—tools with which we can use our inherited capacities while exploring around unknown corners. Today the invention of new devices has become a quest in itself. With their help we seek to discover what further features of our world are "obvious," while remaining to be recognized, measured and put to use.

Earlier centuries gave us field glasses and telescopes with which our eyes can have big images of distant objects and find a wealth of fine detail invisible otherwise. With microscopes our awareness has been extended first into a world in miniature, populated by unbelievable animals and bacteria, and then to the realm of giant molecules. In the last few decades, both vision and hearing have been widened enormously through applications of radio, which resembles light in being free to travel outside the earth's atmosphere, through the vast reaches of the universe. Today we feel less hemmed in by our inborn senses, for tremendous progress during the last five human lifespans has extended our horizons. No final limit, in fact, is in sight for us as we increase our use for the senses we inherit.

I

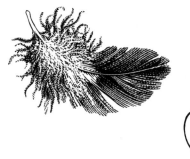

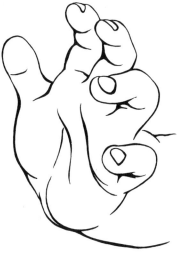

2. *Guiding Touches*

AMONG THE various birds who trust us, whether members of several parrot kinds in the house or wild chickadees coming to our outdoor feeders, we notice a clear distinction between touching and being touched. The chickadee or the lovebird may be willing to rest on a finger and be fed. It may just rest and preen, as though a finger were a branch. Yet the same bird is likely to shy away from an advancing finger, or peck at us if we attempt to stroke its soft breast feathers. It isn't afraid of the finger, for it often hops on and chirps from the new vantage point. The bird merely shows that it doesn't want to be touched. Only a friendly parrot in the right mood will turn its double-hinged beak away, fan out its neck plumage, and invite anyone to rub its head.

Our nervous systems distinguish between touches in the

same way. Those due to our own movements are clearly different from any produced by the activity of something near us. When a man flexes his wrist, or a woman with flowing hair turns her head, many hairs are displaced enough to change the pressures in the skin around the hair follicles. Luckily, we ignore the changes and fail to be disturbed by them. But if a weight of only a thousandth of an ounce be added as a pressure at the end of a hair three-eighths of an inch long, it will bend the bristle as though it were a lever and alert us. We notice immediately if a person or some object touches a hair and bends it, or interferes with its customary bending as we move.

Differences between actively touching things in the environment and passively being touched by them give meaning to the whiskers of a cat or mouse. The long stiff bristles extending from each side of the animal's face excite anyone's curiosity. So, in modern times, does a "handlebar mustache." What are they for? Since all normal cats, mice and men have whiskers, these bristles need not express personality or vanity or cover a scar. They serve, instead, as tactile aids, extending the individual's awareness of the surroundings at times when eyes and ears receive no useful information or are busy with other details.

The prowling cat thrusts her head into a dark hole. Her whiskers graze its sides and inform her of its boundaries. If she brushes against the outstretched quivering bristles of a mouse, the rodent leaps for its life and may reach a place of greater seclusion. But let the mouse blindly touch one of the cat's whiskers or extended eyebrow bristles, and she reacts with the speed and assurance of a mousetrap. Her long hairs are the triggers she depends upon when light and sound and scent are too poor for other sense organs to use. A bearded man might profit too, and learn more from touch in the dark than his baldfaced spouse!

In a muddy stream the catfish relies upon the sense of touch in whiskerlike fleshy barbels which droop toward the bottom and bump into many objects of interest, ones the fish might otherwise miss. The lobster and the crayfish reach out long flexible antennae from their crevices underwater, extending their world of awareness that much farther. Around coral reefs and pilings in tropical seas, the red-

banded barbershop shrimp keeps three pairs of antennae in constant motion. Each of these milk-white, whiplike
appendages is two to three times as long as the animal's
body. It probes the surrounding water like the weaving,
slender beam from a searchlight against the night sky.

Where light from the sun never reaches, whether in a
great cave or the abysses of the seas, animals keep apprised
of their surroundings by means of long extensions from the
body. For every cave cricket flicking its tremendous brown
antennae, the ocean depths have a hundred shrimps and
crabs and squids spreading their feelers and slender legs
and sensitive arms. In this way they improve their chances
of detecting the approach of enemies and of finding food.

In the water world, both salt and fresh, a great variety of
polyps and jellyfishes angle for prey with tentacles as slender as a fisherman's line. Those of the famous Portuguese
man-of-war may trail forty feet into the depths below the
iridescent pinkish-blue float as it drifts before the surface
winds. Each of these fishing lines is studded with special
nettling cells capable of injecting an anesthetic into the
body of any creature small enough to serve as prey, and of
holding it securely until the whole tentacle can contract
and bring the victim to a feeding center.

The flowerlike sea anemones, which decorate rocky
shores but pull in their tentacles when the tide exposes
them to air, wait for the informative touch of a small crab
or a fish swimming against the soft surface of the extended,
petal-like tentacles. Yet even in these seemingly simple
animals, the distinction between active "touching" and
passive "being touched" is evident. Some anemones ride
around on the salvaged snail shells with which hermit
crabs cover the unarmored part of the body. These anemones scarcely contract when they are bumped into
underwater objects in the jerky journeyings of the hermit
crabs they ride. But a shrimp or fish that barely grazes the
outstretched tentacles is seized promptly and devoured.

In some parts of the world, the touch of fish and anemone
shows even more subtle distinctions. In Red Sea waters, at
the marine biological laboratory of Egypt's Fouad I
University, Dr. H. A. F. Gohar found that the common
fish *Amphiprion bicinctus* works in partnership with the

abundant sea anemone *Actinia quadricolor*. Large fish of this kind drive away enemies of the anemones, as though defending their own homes. The anemones, in fact, remain partly contracted unless they receive at frequent intervals the light touch of an *Amphiprion* fish swimming past. Nor does the anemone make any attempt to capture this kind of fish, even when *Amphiprion* takes big bites from some other prey the anemone has caught. Yet, if something pushes an *Amphiprion* into the anemone's tentacles, the sensation is different. The anemone then will seize its "own" fish, sting it and devour it if it is small enough to be engulfed.

For us, touch is seldom so important. Like smell and taste, it can rarely serve as a get-away sense, warning us of danger, or as a means of communication while we are members of a group. Touch, like taste, is so immediate that it may not save us when we are on the brink of disaster. By the time a lion's whiskers graze a person's arm, it is already too late — except for the lion!

Why then, we may wonder, is our sense of touch capable of such exquisite refinement? No special skill is needed to feel the difference between a smooth pane of glass and one etched with grooves 1/2500 of an inch deep. Routinely we take note of surfaces we touch, estimating their hardness or softness, their smoothness or roughness, and whether they are dry, wet, slippery or sticky. Between forefinger and thumb we get an indication of thickness, of stiffness and flexibility. Even a momentary tap with a fingernail against a surface, while our ears are covered to exclude auditory cues, is usually enough to let us identify the material touched as metal, wood, paper, plastic or fabric.

A dry-goods merchant becomes skilled at comparing qualities of cloth by touch. His judgments on this basis are still crude by comparison with those of professional "cloth feelers" in textile houses, whose whole living depends upon the sensitivity in their finger tips. The temptation is to conclude that cloth catches on the friction ridges of human skin and gives the necessary clues to its texture. More than this simple action is involved, however, for a cloth feeler can pursue his trade almost as well after his fingers have been coated with a smooth film of collodion. Many of them can judge a fabric merely by rubbing it with a stick! A tap against the cloth surface, limited to a three-hundredth of a second, has been found adequate to allow complete identification of the material touched.

A quick touch is enough for many kinds of animals too. Ants that stalk springtail insects as prey make the decision whether to seize or reject a springtail too rapidly for the human eye to follow. Eight different kinds of ants with this ability seem to rely upon sensitive hairs projecting from the equivalent of their upper lip—a fringelike moustache. Let these hairs come into contact with a fat-bodied podurid springtail and the ant backs away, utterly avoiding it. But if the hairs touch a more slender entomobryid springtail, the ant's jaws snap convulsively and snatch at the prey. In both of these reactions the ant is far faster than the springtail, despite the fact that these minute creatures are ready at any moment to flick a tail tip and bound abruptly out of reach.

Far slower and easier to trigger is the response to touch in "doodlebugs"—the famous antlions so many children of our southern states discover hiding at the bottom of shallow conical pits of warm sand. While the doodlebug is waiting for a careless ant to run over the rim of the pit, any trivial avalanche of sand grains will get action. The antlion uses its flat head to throw up a rain of sand from the bottom, as though realizing that this will confuse an ant and help it blunder ever closer to the tonglike jaws waiting below. Usually a few seconds suffice to bring a victim into touch with the doodlebug, and the brief, one-sided battle ends.

To start an antlion throwing sand requires just three or four grains of sand. Their combined weight is so small that only a sensitive balance will give an accurate measurement. Yet scientists are interested in such figures, in the amount of energy needed to give a sensation. Nor do they find that touch is as delicate a sense as many of us believe. The best that any person or animal can manage still depends upon receiving from 100 million to 10,000 million times as much energy as is needed for a sensation from the eye or ear.

Touch, moreover, tends to fade out as a stimulus. Unless the skin moves in relation to an object, the feeling disappears completely. Actually, our sensitive nerve endings report only while motion continues, even if this is the short time during which an added weight is sinking slowly by compressing the skin, or while the skin recovers from the slight deformity produced by a weight that has been removed.

To be guided by touch, we must move or wait until we are touched. Animals are similar. Barnacles in their immature swimming stage spend hours or days testing surfaces, finding grooves as attachment sites where they can settle and spend the rest of their lives walled in a self-made limy shell. So too the queen honeybee wanders over the brood comb, reaching her antennae into one cell after another. If the cell is small, she reacts by a nervous reflex that opens a valve in her reproductive system, permitting a few sperm cells to pass through and fertilize an egg; a few minutes later she deposits the egg in the small cell, providing the beginning for another worker bee or a new queen. But if the cell is large, the queen goes right ahead with her laying operation, depositing an unfertilized egg which can develop only into a drone. The sense of touch determines which sex the individual offspring will have.

The reactions of barnacle and bee to the sense of touch depend almost entirely upon inborn features of the nervous system. They are limited in versatility, yet adequate for the usual conditions of life encountered by these creatures. Our experiences in feeling surfaces and spaces can be more cumulative and versatile. No limit may be set to the variety of messages that a person is able to receive through fingers trained to identify raised dots upon a page in the code devised more than a century ago by Louis Braille, the French teacher of the blind. Nor need someone who has learned to use a typewriter "by touch" be able to read Braille in order to communicate with the blind by touch. The typist can use a special typewriter that embosses the code dots upon the page when its keys are pressed in the ordinary fashion. The machine serves to translate visible letters into recognizable protuberances.

A blind person pays better attention to messages received through the sense of touch, and realizes how important this substitute for eyes can be. A few of these handicapped people have noticed that, when some pres-

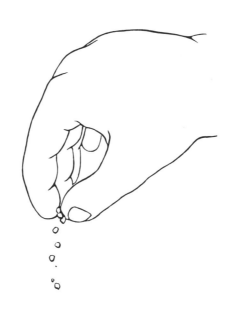
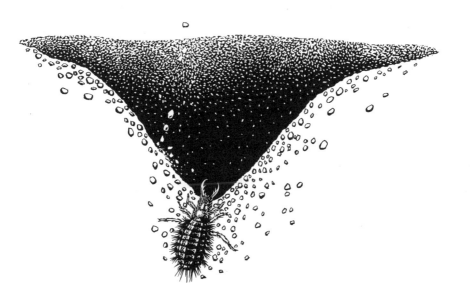

sure on an arm or leg has "put it to sleep," sensitivity to touch and to cold are the first to disappear. They are also the last to reappear as weight is shifted and circulation to the nerves restored. The senses of warmth and ability to feel pain remain active longer and return sooner. With narcotics such as cocaine, however, the sequence differs: pressure is last to be anesthetized, and may even continue while the senses of pain and temperature are dulled into oblivion.

New meanings for the sense of touch have been discovered in recent years. Apparently all of us need to be tousled somewhat, particularly while young. The touch contacts of rough play are essential to development of a normal, friendly personality. Anything short of physical damage seems to have the same effect.

Pet fanciers have known for a long time that the only really tame birds are those that are handled gently and frequently day after day, almost from the time they hatch. Yet scientific proof of this need for touch came only in the last decade when infant rats were tested in a novel way. One third of the experimental animals were left in the nests, unhandled. Another third of them were lifted carefully by hand into special boxes and kept there for many minutes at a time, several times a day. The final third were placed in similar boxes but subjected to mildly painful electric shocks for the same number of minutes on the identical schedule.

No symptoms of neurosis or other abnormal behavior appeared among the shocked rats as they matured. The animals subjected to stress by electric stimulation were just as friendly as those that had been transferred to boxes and kept there. Instead, it was the "control group" of rats —those left unhandled in the nests—that showed a difference. These nonmanipulated animals, as they grew up, crept timidly about or cowered in a corner, showing their anxiety by eliminating wastes at frequent intervals. At maturity, they reacted to brain surgery eliminating fear in a way never encountered before, becoming "the most excitable and vicious rats" ever observed. The handled rats, after similar surgery, remained comparatively tame.

Psychiatrists see a parallel between the nonmanipulated

infant rats left well fed and warm in the nests and the human child in a foundling home where fondling is at a minimum. Perhaps the rats answered the old question of whether to spank or not to spank. Certainly the infant rats subjected to painful electric shocks received no explanation for the punishment. Yet they developed normally, without antagonisms toward the experimenters. They were far better off than the rats that received no individual handling.

At the University of Wisconsin, Dr. Harry F. Harlow and his colleagues have been pressing this intriguing question another step. What is mother love, and how is it engendered? To learn the answers, they have been taking newborn macaque monkeys from their mothers and caging them at the age of two days with a substitute ("surrogate") parent of approximately correct size, fitted with a single nipple from which warm milk can be taken at any time. One type of substitute mother has a body of chicken wire. The other consists of a wooden cylinder wrapped in sponge rubber and clad in terry cloth. Both surrogate parents wear rotatable wooden heads with buttons or reflectors in place of eyes, and are supported from the floor at an angle, slanting backward.

The infant monkeys soon discover the nipple and nurse when hungry. But only the soft, cloth-covered "mother" engenders the affectional responses a person would describe as "baby love." The little monkey with the chicken-wire "mother" goes to "her" only for food, as a customer might seek out the little glass door at the Automat. It does not go to "her" when confronted with some terrifying object, but cowers instead in a corner, screaming and trying to hide under its own arms. By contrast, an infant monkey with a soft "mother" spends much of its time hugging her, twisting her head around and around, perching on her armless shoulders. "She" is a constant comfort, a "mother" whose patience never becomes exhausted, and a refuge to which the monkey infant rushes when a terrifying object is presented. Even in this response a difference is evident: the infant seems to soak up confidence from the cloth-covered "parent," and soon becomes curious enough to venture toward the terrifying object and examine it—at first briefly, and then without hesitation.

A newborn macaque is more mature at birth than is a human baby, but its responses relating to affection and exploration of its world show no striking differences. It grows more rapidly and develops in a few weeks many of the habits that a human child needs months to acquire. Both depend extensively upon the sense of touch in building personalities.

Our modern society tends to provide a nursing bottle and canned baby food as a substitute for a mother's breast, and to free the female parent for gainful employment at a machine, or for welfare work, or for self-centered pleasure of many kinds. It is encouraging to see scientific evidence showing that a man, displaced from earning the family's living, can serve just as well as his spouse in giving his children what they need for normal mental growth. He may not bear the babies, but they can find his heavy touch as love-inducing as her lighter one would be.

So far we have not met much success with extending and improving our sense of touch. If we want to measure something with greater accuracy than a machinist's fingers can achieve with a micrometer reading to a ten-thousandth of an inch, we bypass touch and enlarge the part optically to let us make a visual comparison. Almost the only invention in which a passive counterpart of touch is turned to good advantage takes the form of machines that handle punched cards, identify the coded holes, and take appropriate action. One card with its many holes, unmoving in the machine, is enough to give information. Depending upon the "sophistication" of the machine—actually the cleverness with which an engineer has laid out the circuits in its electrical viscera—the device can do routine work, often far faster than a person.

To be replaced by a punch-card machine is no compliment to anyone's sensory abilities and mental co-ordination, for no machine with an electric circuit in lieu of a brain can show the versatility and sensitivity of a man. As soon as the device suffers an internal breakdown or meets a punch card with some combination of holes for which no programming has been arranged, the best the machine can do is to turn on a red light, stop, and wait for a skillful technician to rescue it. Otherwise it will make mistakes we would never forgive in an alert human being.

Fortunately, touch coupled with continued motion is something different, and more open to engineering development. The difference is as simple as the stylus resting quietly in a groove of a phonograph record with the machine stopped, and the same juxtaposition with the disc rotating. Touch plus continued motion can give meaningful vibrations, both in an instrument and in an animal's body. But touch alone still challenges us to exploit it.

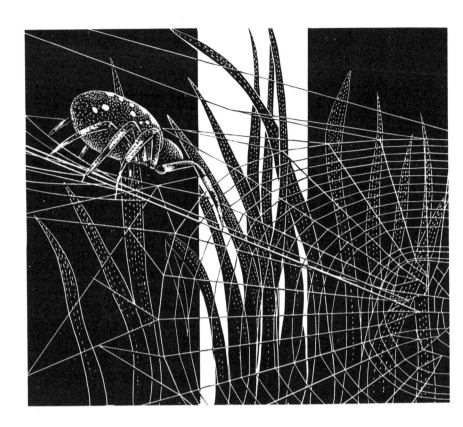

3. *The Languages of Vibration*

How MANY of us have reached out a finger to a sleeping house cat and tickled the hairs fringing an ear? The ear twitches, without the animal awakening. Or we have used a blade of grass to stroke the bare skin on a pad of the cat's foot, inducing the pet to shake its whole leg. If either of these gentle disturbances continues, the cat will rouse itself to see what is going on.

Our own response to tickling varies greatly. When we are in deep sleep, the sole of a foot can be stroked with a feather time after time without bringing any reaction. In lighter slumber, we withdraw the foot from the feather, without awakening or remembering afterward. Yet, when fully alert, the same stimulation can be sheer torture and, if prolonged, can induce hysterics.

Movement is the feature we notice. Let an insect weighing half as much as an appleseed alight on the bare back of a sunbather. If it merely takes two steps, then flies away, the spot where it touched down has been vibrated, shaken ever so gently. The skin there may itch until scratched with vigor. Yet an appleseed, dropped on the same site, would be noticed for only a moment, then ignored and forgotten because it stayed still.

Despite careful study by many able scientists, we do not yet know for sure whether human sensitivity to vibrations in the skin arises from the unspecialized endings of fine nerves reaching into the outside layer, or is due to a multiplicity of more complex sense organs in underlying levels. Scientists are as well aware as lock pickers that the outer horny, dead portions of the skin reduce our sensitivity by absorbing some of the energy from vibrant stimuli. Lock pickers have long been known to use sandpaper before a burglary job, to remove the dead outermost skin over their finger tips until the slight and inaudible jar of a metal tumbler in a lock can be sensed, yielding clues to the combination for a safe.

Our finger tips excel in their acuity to vibrations. They tell us how long a quiver lasts, what vigor it shows, and something of its rate of motion. The palm of the hand and the sole of the foot inform us nearly as well. So do the lips. But, as we age, the finger tips retain their acuity almost unimpaired, whereas other parts of the body decline in sensitivity.

These abilities in detecting vibrations are actually an exquisite refinement of touch—a recognition that the area of a pressure has changed. The pulsations may remain centered at the same point, but be noticed as alternating increases and decreases in the area pressed upon. Or the region of pressure may shift sidewise at less than a snail's pace and be sensed because of its movement.

Communications engineers and psychologists have often wondered how our skin's sensitivity to vibration might be put to fuller use. Certainly we neglect most of its possibilities. Even the area available for receiving messages is impressive. A woman of ordinary size has about fifteen square feet of surface, and her mate as much as twenty-three. This is more than a thousand times as large a surface as the light-sensitive retinas of the two eyes combined, and ten thousand times the total area of the two eardrums. Yet we use our skins chiefly as radiators for body heat, and lose through them daily a considerable amount of moisture.

Curiously enough, our chilled skins are more sensitive to vibrations of all kinds than when warm. A warm skin lets us be more aware than a cool one of pressures that do not move or vibrate. Since the same receptor system appears to advise us of both vibrations and steady pressure, the temperature difference in our sensitivity to each must be due to changes in the flexibility of the skin.

Our greatest sensitivity to vibrations lies in the range of audible sounds, between two hundred and one hundred vibrations per second. The ear detects air vibrations of these rates as corresponding to G♯ below middle C on the piano keyboard and the next G♯ lower still. The lowest registers of a tenor voice and of a cello fall between these two. What could be more normal, then, than for a scientist to inquire whether a person might not be taught to "hear" through his skin—interpreting words or sentences transmitted entirely as vibrations against a finger tip or the chest wall or the surface of a thigh?

At Northwestern University, the psychologist Dr. R. H. Gault made such an attempt in the early 1920's. Against the fingers he applied the vibrations from human speech, suitably amplified. The person who served as the "feeler" in the experiment learned, after twenty-eight half-hour training sessions, to judge correctly three times out of four which of ten short sentences had been vibrated against the fingers. Single words out of context were much harder to identify even after long practice. And if the speaker changed his rate of talking, or someone else said the same words, the "feeler" became hopelessly confused.

Recently, new hopes have been raised for training people to use the neglected vibratory sense in their skins. Although the methods are still experimental, some of the results are highly encouraging. It is just as easy, for example, to signal silently to an airplane pilot or a racing-car driver that it is time to turn left or right by a vibratory message applied to his chest skin as to tell him the same thing by means of flashing lights or words through his ears. Skin messages, in fact, come through clearly when the ears are all but deafened by continuous loud noise, and in complete darkness.

One way to give these vibratory messages is to fasten to the skin with tape small vibrators that can be driven electrically. If a person wears one on the right side, another on the left, and if the right one vibrates a few tenths of a second before an identical signal is felt on the left, the illusion is one of a buzzing that travels to the left—a signal to turn left. Vibrators high and low on the midline of the chest are just as suitable for directing a pilot to nose his aircraft up or down. A set of four vibrators can bring him instructions relating to adjustments needed in both the horizontal and vertical planes. They provide no serious distraction for eyes and ears and are as intimate as a tap on the shoulder. Nor does the brain become confused over remembering which side is right.

At the University of Virginia, where these explorations of skin messages have been in progress since the late 1950's, a brand-new sensation has been discovered. If six vibrators are stuck to the skin in an imaginary ring around the torso—three on the chest and three on the back—and these are buzzed in a quick sequence for a fraction of a second apiece, the brain interprets the vibratory message as a vivid swirling that is continuous and "completely prepossessing." It is something like an electrical hula hoop spinning without effort.

Professor Frank A. Geldard, who directs these studies, regards the swirling stimulus as a perfect way to alert a person when a general alarm button is pressed. It is a signal of universal application, independent of language, age, sex, occupation and possible handicap such as blindness or deafness. It cannot be confused with any other signal, yet it demands immediate attention.

No one would particularly relish the idea of wearing a string of vibrators and a radio pickup as a warning system. But a fashion expert could incorporate such a device into a money belt or even the top part of a Bikini bathing suit. It might be linked silently to an electronic babysitter, translating the child's cry into a message felt privately by one or both parents. The father, who never experienced a kick from within by his unborn child, could suddenly feel himself surrounded by a whirling vibration each time the baby howled. This reminder of responsibility might reach him at a poker game or on a tavern stool, and send him hurrying home to change the child.

For many years now, therapists have been teaching the deaf to communicate by finger signals. Many have learned to interpret these entirely by touch, a feat that opened the world to Helen Keller and others like her who lack both sight and hearing. Is this language of the fingers the most efficient means for transmitting information by touch? Need the hands be involved at all, or could they be employed gainfully at other tasks while the messages reach unused areas of the skin?

The group of scientists at the University of Virginia have attacked these problems too. Dr. W. C. Howell devised a simple alphabetic code that can be learned more easily than Braille. It matches a person's ability to recognize which of three vibrators on the chest—a right, a center and a left—is buzzed, and to judge among three different intensities of stimulation, and to distinguish among three unlike lengths of signal, of which the briefest lasts a mere tenth of a second. One student, who cooperated by spending thirty hours learning the code and an additional thirty-five hours of training in its use, was able to understand with 90 per cent accuracy whole sentences received as vibrations transmitted to him at the rate of thirty-eight five-letter words per minute. This is one and a half times as fast as the speed of radio operators proficient in the Morse code. Further practice with the Howell type of "vibratese" would reach a theoretical ceiling rate of 67 five-letter words per minute, "a speed well over three times that of proficient Morse." The bottleneck now, in fact, is the engineering job needed to produce a machine able to send messages so fast. Fingers will not tap out the code as fast as any human skin area can receive it and the brain perform the translation!

Whatever the future of vibratory messages to human

body surfaces, it is clear that we are barely beginning to explore a sense already used extensively by other animals. From them we could learn a great deal. For far too long we have ignored the vibrations our bare feet might pick up from the ground when an annoyed skunk stamps a warning, before using his malodorous spray.

Lock makers could profit from understanding insects more thoroughly. The last few years have brought proof that these most numerous of all kinds of creatures cooperate in mating only when each partner presses the other at definite spots sensitive to vibration. The number and pattern of these areas differ from one species to the next. They are the secret buttons that take the place of locks and keys in safeguarding the reproductive purity of each insect species. With nearly 700,000 kinds of insects already recognized and hundreds more being discovered annually, the number of combinations seems almost endless.

Some animal responses to vibration add refinements to normal behavior. No special sensitivity is needed to keep an insect facing into the wind or moving toward it; the animal maintains its balance more easily while doing so than while traveling in any other direction. But vibration-sensitive organs within the third joint of a blowfly's antennae allow the insect to judge when the wind rises to 1.6 miles per hour. At this critical wind velocity the insect stops flying. These creatures are now known to possess a whole series of sensitive areas along the leading edge of each thin wing. They seem to use them as part of the control needed in flight. Air flowing over the wing edge sets up vibrations in the sense organs, informing the nervous system and letting it order the correct muscular contractions to adjust the wings' camber and attack angle in each cycle of beating.

Honeybees, standing on the surface of the hive, are so sensitive to vibrations reaching them through their feet that they can be distracted and lose all concern for the welfare of the colony and its honey stores. The most effective vibrations are those matching sounds from one to two octaves above the standard A pitch to which musicians tune their instruments when they come on stage. A buzzing device which could be attached temporarily to the side of a hive was recommended in 1956 as a tool useful in im-mobilizing bees while harvesting their honey. It was surer than smoke, and did not hurt the insects in any way.

Within the dark hive, honeybees are particularly sensi-tive to the nudges and vibrations they receive from recently returned workers, who dance out a message on the vertical surface of the comb and tell the distance and direction to the nectar source from which they have been collecting. Communication of this kind is lacking, however, in the stingless social bees of the genus *Trigona*, found in the tropics and warm countries. They give no dances, respond to no nudging and vibrations on the honeycomb, and are far less efficient at learning where to go for more food as workers return.

If scientists had any lingering doubts that the nudging dances and vibratory language of the bees were real, these misgivings vanished in early 1959 when Dr. Wolfgang Steche of Munich demonstrated his ability to communi-cate as a honeybee does. He equipped a working hive with an artificial bee whose dances on the comb surface he could control remotely by electronic means. With levers he manipulated his artificial bee on unseen dances inside the hive, "telling" live bees that crowded around the imitation insect where to go for nectar. Within a few minutes a whole stream of bees headed straight for a food supply set out for them—sugar water no bee had visited previously.

Honeybees use their nudging dances also on a very different occasion. After a swarm emerges from the hive and hangs up in a mass around the old queen, the majority of the bees wait quietly until their scouts have located a number of prospective sites. Each returning scout performs her dance on the surface of the swarm, and a few more bees go off to investigate the place communicated to them. The excitement of the investigators, when they arrive back at the swarm, is related to the suitability of the site they have examined. Gradually this excitement spreads, and all of the bees that have been on hole-hunting expeditions begin to dance in one direction. Only then does the whole swarm respond, departing for its new home, clearly con-vinced when the scouts are unanimous.

Vibrations serve the communication needs of a great variety of animals. The web of a spider is a telegraph line whose gentle shaking tells her through special sense organs on her legs how big a fly has blundered into her trap. If it is too small, she may ignore it. If the vibrations are violent, she is likely to rush out and cut the victim loose, thereby saving the rest of her net. Or she may cower in a corner until a big beetle breaks free and leaves her the task of rebuilding the whole web. Only a middle-sized vibration means food to her, and sends her scurrying to wrap it up.

Male spiders of web-weaving kinds often engage in web twitching, ascertaining in this way the degree of hunger in a potential mate. If the female is hungry, the vibrations of her running on the web warn the male to flee for his life. If she merely signals that she is home, he is likely to advance a few steps at a time. Lucky males father a new generation of spiderings and escape again before it is too late.

In water, vibrations can be even more meaningful by bringing news of events at a distance. On spring nights, when salamanders return to the ponds of their youth to swim and mate, they depend upon detecting faint pulsations in the dark water. Before the male will respond to vibrations, however, his mating instinct must be released by the flavor of females of his own kind in the pond. Then he will approach any swimmer as a potential mate. That the vibrations are not specific messages is shown by male salamanders that will hurry toward even a slowly swimming fish, finding it by the slight agitation of the water generated by its heart and movements of its gills, fins and tail.

Fishes too depend upon vibrations. Only our inability to sense these cues through our skins as water animals do keeps us from knowing how widespread these habits are. Size cannot guide us, since the two-inch stickleback and the forty-inch salmon both follow mating routines based upon sensitivity to a quivering mate who is not in actual contact. In each instance the female will not lay her eggs until she feels this vibration or some substitute. Indian guides know that a canoe paddle, jarred rapidly while dipped into the water, can often fool an unaccompanied female salmon into laying. A glass rod vibrated close to the tail of a female stickleback has the same effect if she is ready to deposit her eggs.

In the light of day, as we watch by a pond or a winding stream, it is easy to regard the water as though it were a window display behind glass. We do not expect it to affect any human sense except vision. If we think of vibratory messages in the water at all, we tend to regard as totally unlike ourselves any animal that depends naturally upon information sensed through its body surface. Yet a toad whose reproductive hormones are so like our own that it is used world-wide in tests for human pregnancy at early stages fits this other pattern of sensitivity. It is the African clawed toad *Xenopus,* raised by the thousands in aquaria today, for it remains aquatic throughout life. As an adult its sides bear a set of vibration-sensitive organs somewhat resembling those in the lateral line canal of fishes. With these organs the African toad can locate an insect or other moving object that could serve as prey, even in the most turbid water and at distances up to four inches.

Wild creatures found in almost any pond can do as well or better, although we have watched some of them countless times without realizing this. The backswimmer insect *Notonecta* sometimes is so close below the water film that we can see its beak, on the upper surface because the creature lives upside down. This insect's coloration matches its strange position, and camouflages the half-inch stream-lined body. The backswimmer rows along while seeking bees or other insects that fall into the pond, and relies upon vibrations produced by its struggling prey. A back-swimmer can detect them night or day, at six inches distant or even more. Now when we see this bug poised an inch or two below the surface, with its long pair of sculling legs outstretched and motionless, we know that it is alert—not sleeping.

Some of our commonest water insects find still more refined uses for vibrations in the water. The many kinds of glossy black whirligig beetles detect ripples of their own making, when these are reflected from the shore, from obstacles in their path or from the sides of an aquarium tank. As a whirligig zigs and zags on the surface of ponds and slow streams anywhere in the world, it senses these reflected ripples by means of its antennae floating in the surface film, supported there by a fringe of special hairs. Between each swimming dash and the next, the whirligig coasts and is alert to meaning in every wavelet. If its antennae are cemented to the head and cannot serve the insect in this way, it blunders into everything and seems unable to find food floating on the surface. Even by day it needs its vibration-sensitive antennae if it is to match its darting to the quick maneuvers of its fellow beetles. Apparently its eyes do not provide accurate information fast enough for such split-second decisions.

It is hard for us to think of any sense as being better than eyes by day. Yet all sorts of animals with sensitive skins and body surfaces show us that for them the language of vibrations is more meaningful. For millions of years they have been developing their special sensitivities, whereas for us the whole idea of messages through our skins is still quite new. Can we meet the challenge of adapting these abilities to our own purposes? Should we overlook any avenue for communication from a distance? If we choose to put vibratory sense to work for us, we should be able to do so, and to regard the outcome as progress.

Progress itself has a paradoxical quality. The noises of civilization match progress: monster trucks, pneumatic tools, powerful public address systems and jet aircraft. If their deafening sounds double again in intensity, as they have in the recent past, we may all need to wear protective ear stopples and give up trying to talk to one another. Perhaps then our skins will serve best for mass communication. Only minor modifications are needed to convert a transistor radio in the shirt pocket into a device communicating silently in vibratory code. It is tempting to wonder what international code might be agreed upon.

Communication with other animals is also within reach today, through vibratory code. Fewer bees and fewer man hours would be needed in achieving full pollination of America's orchard trees if the methods of automation were extended to directing these insects in the way we now know how to follow. Today, trucks with beehives are contracted for, to travel from orchard to orchard and bring bees when the apples or peaches are in flower. The bees are often supplied, at the doorway to each hive, with a trough full of the proper pollen. They have to wade through it while emerging to fly away, and thus are ready to pollinate every fruit-tree flower they reach. Each truck could carry, in addition, an electronic device linked to imitation bees mounted on the honeycombs, as models that would dance according to a program supplied by a technician. An observant man, cruising just above the fruit trees in a light airplane, could send radio messages to the technician aboard the truck, informing him which blocks of trees were just opening their flowers and ready for bees. The technician could type on his special tape machine the dance instructions for the imitation bees, and load the troughs with pollen. Each live bee would head in the prescribed direction, without needing to wait for scouts to return with samples. Days might be saved, and the still-uncontrolled weather dodged more efficiently. All of this is perfectly feasible without delay.

Today we tend toward ever more automation, relegating man to a supervisory role. We save our senses and ingenuity for meeting emergencies. At the same time, we try to anticipate each possibility and prepare for it. This might be regarded as the present stage in human evolution. The earliest step may well have been the one conjectured by Harvard University's philosopher-entomologist William Morton Wheeler. According to his view, a sudden genetic change occurred in one group of anthropoid apes about a million years ago. The affected individuals showed a new dominant passion: to improve everything, to progress. This ancestral line led to mankind. Somewhere along the way, the descendants must have lost interest in vibrations through the skin. Perhaps we now need to make up for lost time. By alerting ourselves again to vibratory cues, we may even emerge with a fresh awareness of our world.

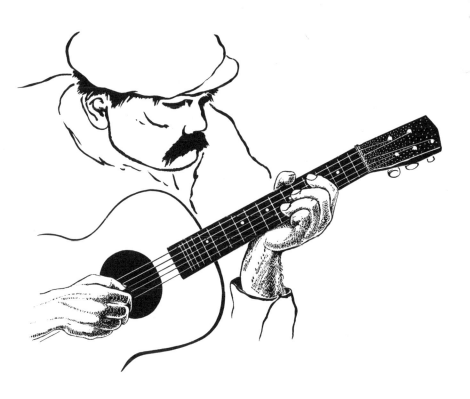

What Do Ears Tell Us?

WITHIN THE earth's atmosphere, almost everything makes a sound. Lightning leaps from soil to cloud and heats the air in its path into such explosive expansion that a shock wave rushes away "at the speed of sound," as a clap of thunder.

Thunder used to terrify each of us. We still stay alert whenever an electrical storm is in our vicinity, but at least our minds are eased by a little game our parents taught us. If we count the seconds between each flash of lightning and its matching clap of thunder, then divide the total by five, we learn how many miles away the lightning struck. Most storms pass by without coming closer than a mile. Only when the flash and the thunderclap arrive together is there danger, for in air at ordinary temperatures, one second is needed for sound to travel eleven hundred feet. If there's no time to count, you're hit!

On the sea beach, we've found more relaxed pleasure in counting the crash of waves, judging their size by the loudness of the noise, and wondering how true is the claim that every ninth wave is larger than those between. Or we can realize, while sunbathing, how distinctive the repetitious sounds can be: the boom of breakers against a rocky coast, the "grating roar of pebbles" Matthew Arnold described on the beach below the cliffs of Dover, the shard-like clatter of disturbed shell fragments along some tropical shore, or the hissing escape of air from sand overflowed by quieter invasions of the waves in a protected bay.

Anyone who presses his ear against the beach can hear the thud of each wave's impact before the sound reaches him through the air, for the vibrations travel almost ten times as rapidly through the more substantial earth. The wary Bushmen in Africa's great Kalahari Desert know how much better the soil serves as a conductor of sound. These primitive people invariably sleep on their sides, literally with one ear to the ground and the other fully exposed to the air. Usually the man lies on his left side and the wife on her right, facing her husband across the little fire that helps keep them warm through the chilly night. In this way they have a better chance to detect the approach of an animal while the information can still be useful.

Perhaps most sounds in nature are incidental to activity of some kind. It is doubtful that any creature save man finds pleasure in them. Surely this is a measure of our gain. We can attune our ears to leaves vibrated by the wind, and compare the sound with others we have heard. The clatter of living palm fronds in a tropical breeze becomes indistinguishable from the pelt of rain on dry, dead leaves on a temperate forest floor. The multitude of twittering green triangles in an aspen, a cottonwood or a poplar may simulate the riffle in a brook, where the water breaks in wavelets over the stones. For Mary Webb, wind-blown grass possessed "the very voice of Earth." Yet poets have no monopoly on these pleasures; they merely help others become aware of them. Anyone can appreciate the soft whisper of air flowing between the fine needles of a Maine pine, or the fanning of the blades in a Canadian maple. Each tree has a voice of its own.

What fisherman does not gladden to the splash of a fish falling back into the water after a lusty leap into air? What horseman fails to find companionship in the nose-clearing snort of his steed browsing at night in the dew-wet grass? The hum of bees in an apple tree is a song of spring, and the whirr of a hummingbird's wings before a flower a sign of summer weather. None of these is deliberate communication. Their meaning for us is limited largely by what our eyes have seen beforehand.

Even when we can credit a sound with having been produced by an animal in response to some stimulus, it is not always safe to assume that the vibrations have meaning for the animal itself or for others of its kind. John R. Pierce and Edward E. Davis, Jr., tell of an acquaintance who became intrigued with the apparent unison with which crickets chirped in a New Jersey meadow. He built an electronic chirp maker whose sound seemed a reasonably good imitation, although its pitch and rate of chirp repetition could both be adjusted over a wide range. With a couple of colleagues for company he took the device in his station wagon along the highway to a place where crickets could be heard plainly, and there the three men started to set up the equipment. First a suspicious state highway patrolman made them move on. But eventually they found a suitable site and made their tests. No matter how they adjusted the instrument, the crickets ignored its sounds. Only much later did the baffled men learn from an English expert on crickets that these insects communicate in a sound band high in the ultrasonic range—far above anything audible to man. The "natural" chirps detected by human ears are purely incidental to the ultrasonic notes produced simultaneously by the scraping action of the insects' wings. The experimenters' equipment had emitted only tremendously loud chirps in a range of pitches with no meaning for the crickets.

As adults our sound spectrum extends from about 20 to 20,000 vibrations per second—a range of nearly ten octaves, each a doubling of the vibration rate. Often the acoustic engineer considers the repetitive nature of sound-producing vibrations as cycles, and speaks of "cycles per second" (c.p.s.) instead of the vibrations themselves. As children our ears probably respond to 40,000 c.p.s. But as we grow older, the eardrum gradually thickens and the linkage of the tiny bones transmitting vibrations from drum to the inner ear becomes more resistant to passage of high-frequency sounds. Measurements of men in their forties show that the upper limit of the ear's sensitivity falls about 80 c.p.s. every six months, curtailing our appreciation of the overtones in fine music at a regular, almost sinister rate.

Perhaps this explains why we cling to "middle C" at 256 c.p.s. as a landmark in the musical scale, although it is well below the middle of the audible range, as well as of the piano keyboard and of the full reach of human voices. Around 3,000 c.p.s. is a far more important range of pitches for mankind. There. between F♯ and G in the fourth octave above middle C, we are most sensitive to sound. At this pitch and near it we require least energy in a sound for it to stimulate the ear and give us a sensation. To this is due the "piercing" quality of a scream from a woman or child. A call for help at 3,000 c.p.s. retains audible vibrations farther before it is absorbed by the air and by obstacles. It impresses us as being louder.

From more than an octave below middle C up to the 3,000-c.p.s. level. our hearing and that of a cat are about equal. But the cat's ears respond far more sensitively than ours do to sounds of higher pitch. At 13,000 c.p.s. in the highest octave an ordinary adult human ear will detect, a cat needs only a thousandth as much energy as a man to identify the presence of vibrations. Yet the cat's hearing may not permit the animal to detect the calls of mice pitched even higher. One mouse can hear the warning scream of another, even at moderate intensity, up to 100,000 c.p.s. How much farther up the scale a mouse can hear, or what sounds exist at these high levels, remain as mysteries awaiting the invention of more sensitive microphones able to pick up the ultra-fast vibrations.

One of our graduate students built a sound-translating device with which he could hear for each moderately high-pitched inaudible sound a reasonably low-pitched (and hence audible) substitute. After we had helped him test it by listening to the calls of captive bats and the surprising ultrasonic jingling that accompanies the shaking of a bunch of keys, he took the instrument to the room housing the rat colony belonging to the psychology department. There he discovered that, while the rats are playing games right after they are fed and they open their mouths as though ready to bite one another, they are screaming at the top of their voices—around 24,000 c.p.s. Subsequently he took his electronic translator to the National Zoological Park in Washington and listened to many kinds of mammals. Each had its own communication band—its specific frequency and wave length—with few exceptions.

If each sound-producing animal communicates with others of its kind at a special pitch to which its ears are most sensitive, a call need not be above the intensity of a whisper to be effective. Such a faint sound would be inaudible to most other kinds of animals, since their hearing would not be keenest at the same frequency. Privacy would be assured for each species. Good news and bad could be shared, warnings given and received, without disclosing the location of the individual producing the sound. Matched voices and ears can have great value in survival, even though our appreciation of this fact has been slow to come because of the limitations in our own sensitivity.

No ear could benefit by being ten times as sensitive as ours is at 3,000 c.p.s. Greater sensitivity would, in fact, make the organ respond to the random movement of air molecules. Every louder sound would then be heard against a background hiss—a "white noise" consisting of a great assortment of different rates of vibration without meaning. As it is, when the eardrum responds to the faintest sound we can hear, it moves back and forth a mere forty billionths of an inch—about a tenth the diameter of the smallest atom. Yet the lever action of the three little bones in the middle ear reduces even this minuscule motion while transforming the small pressure of sound on the surface of the eardrum into a 22-fold greater pressure on the fluid enclosed in the inner ear.

The relative insensitivity of the human ear at low frequencies of vibration is important in protecting us from distraction by the vibrations of our own bodies. Merely by stoppering each ear with a finger tip, shutting out airborne sounds, we can detect a pulsating hum given off by the contraction of muscle cells in our fingers and arms.

This simple change, made by blocking the access of airborne sound waves to the eardrums, can be used to show that another route is available to us for the vibrations we hear. When we hum with our lips closed, we largely bypass the eardrum and the tiny bones of the middle ear. The sound is conducted to the inner ear through the skull itself. The sound is louder, in fact, if we hum with ear stopples or even with our fingers closing the canals of the outer ears. Vibrations reaching the eardrum's inner surface, by way of the Eustachian tube from the throat, are then no longer able to pass out through our ears; instead, they are reflected back toward the inner ear and reinforce the bone-conducted sound.

Old violinists, when tuning their instruments, sometimes compensate for the aging of their eardrums and the ear-bone linkages by touching their teeth to the vibrating fiddle. So long as the bony skull will conduct the high notes and let the musician hear them clearly, he knows that he suffers only from transmission deafness. A hearing aid could help him, by applying the amplified vibrations to the head surface just behind the ear. But if this test fails, his ears are probably showing deterioration of the auditory nerve itself, a process for which there is no known remedy. How many other animals suffer from transmission deafness is a mystery. Comparatively few in the wild survive into old age unless their faculties remain exceptionally youthful.

Most of us reserve the gesture of stoppering our ears with finger tips for situations where we want to block out background noise. The rustle of leaves or papers, the steady beating of rain on the roof, the chatter of a large roomful of animated people, the whirr of machines even as simple as a hair dryer, all lead us to raise our voices in pitch and intensity, in an effort to be heard. Yet the energy in the human sounds remains principally in vibratory rates slower than 1,000 c.p.s., no matter whether the voice is that of a man, woman or child. No ordinary talk makes much use of the part of the audible spectrum to which our ears are most sensitive. Seemingly we leave that channel open, as though reserved for emergencies—for any high-pitched scream.

Distinguishing between plain "white" noises is seldom easy. Only experience led us to be amused at the question asked by our neighbor's five-year-old when he came to our front door on a sunny day and heard hamburgers sizzling in the kitchen. His jaw dropped. Then he recovered his amazement and inquired politely, "Is it raining at your back door?" How long has it taken us to learn the difference between the sound of blasting—creating a new gash in New England granite for some foundation or pipeline—and the double boom of a passing jet plane that is exceeding the speed of sound and leaving a great V-shaped shock wave in its wake? Friends tell us that, although no windows near by have been broken yet by the forceful vibrations, many of the new houses going up are designed with no plastered walls or ceilings that a sonic boom could crack.

To a remarkable degree we hear what we expect to hear, whether this is words we know or music stored in our brains as complex sound patterns. From these learned patterns we draw guidance in forming our speech. We listen unconsciously to our own voices and carefully adjust them in relation to this mental pattern.

People who claim accident insurance for having lost their hearing are now tested in a device that delivers through earphones a delayed playback of their own speech. No person who makes a false claim can continue to talk if his ears hear his own words after a delay of two or three tenths of a second; he becomes confused and shows that he is malingering. A truly deaf person is unaffected, and continues to talk as he learned to do before his loss of hearing.

No electronic machine is needed to distinguish between expert and amateur musicians on the basis of what their ears tell them. The expert regulates his touch upon the instrument through even the most difficult passages according to the reverberations of the room in which he is playing. The amateur becomes too engrossed to notice.

For more than a century, teachers of vocal music have stressed the importance of training each singer to produce a vibrato rather than a steady note. This is actually a tremor or warbling change in pitch, over a range of perhaps five to six cycles per second. It is sufficiently pleasing to the human ear that the complexity of a pipe organ is usually increased by a device that mimics vibrato. But in 1959 scientists at Oxford University discovered that the vibrato is essential in controlling one's own singing voice and keeping to an intended pitch. Without the stimulation of the deliberate variation, the singer's brain does not notice gradual changes in key.

Music is a heritage we receive throughout life, from lullaby to symphony. We learn its phrasing, its sequences of tones, until we know what to expect next. Some people rebel against this, and enjoy being teased by the unexpected in music. For this reason they listen to jazz, an American art form specializing in avoiding the "musical clichés" by extensive improvisations that defy the listener to hum the tune a few phrases in advance of what his ears are hearing. This is the essence of "jazzing it up."

The degree to which the human brain is ready to continue a musical cliché is easy to test. We often do so unintentionally when a combination of some well-loved musical work on the radio, a jet plane passing low over the house, and a visitor at the door leads one of us to switch off the music and answer the bell. If this happens when the noise from the plane is overpoweringly loud, the other of us keeps on reading or working, mentally continuing to "hear" the music until the plane is almost out of earshot. Then, suddenly, comes the realization that the radio is silent and a conversation is going on in the living room.

We use learned, memorized patterns in sound also when breaking the flow of vibrations from another person's speech into meaningful pieces. By the time a child is five or six and starting to school, he has spent more than twenty thousand hours learning to interpret by ear the talk of his parents and associates. Perhaps ten thousand complex sequences of syllables have become recognizable, related to events in his surroundings. If more than one language is used routinely at home, the number may be higher. Yet other languages remain "foreign," lacking the familiar "phonemes" in meaningful sequence. Consequently, comparable lengths of time may be needed to add another language with as full appreciation for nuances of meaning and tone of expression.

Other animals differ only in degree in their ability to learn languages. Parrots have become famous in this direction. But does a parrot really recognize more than a certain sequence of pitch changes and five breaks between syllables when somebody asks, "Polly want a cracker?" We had always been doubtful, until that day in South Africa when we were shown a big cageful of handsome *Amazona* parrots confiscated months before from a cargo ship at a port in the Union without proper papers for them.

We like parrots, and asked to be let go into the cage with them, although our host assured us that these birds were far from friendly. He had made countless overtures to them, talking to them in Afrikaans and in English while trying to buy their confidence with gifts of food. Still they remained suspicious and elusive.

Our experiences with *Amazona* parrots have been chiefly in Central America and Mexico, where any tame parrot is *loro* unless you know it to be a female (*lora*) or want to be affectionate by using the diminutive *lorito*. There they are particularly fond of *masa*, the crushed whole soaked corn from which tortillas are made. On the floor of the African cage we saw some rain-soaked corn, and automatically picked it up, mashing it between thumb and forefinger. We held it out and talked to the caged birds in our best Spanish, "Loritos bonitos, comed la masa, la masa sabrosa. Lorito, lorito!" And what did the expatriate *Amazonas* do? They flew to the bar beside us, constricting their golden pupils in excitement, spreading their tails, ruffling the feathers on the backs of their necks, echoing *lorito* over and over in obvious delight. Of course they would eat out of our hands and let us scratch behind their heads! It was so good to hear Spanish again! We had to teach the Afrikaner enough for him to be accepted too.

For a bird to imitate human speech is no proof of its intelligence, of course. We have at least as much reason to suspect that parrots can be taught to "talk" because their own vocal mechanisms and hearing operate more slowly than those of other birds. Human sounds may simply resemble parrot squawks more than the musical repertoire of songbirds.

Probably the brain of any animal pays attention to only a narrow selection from among the sounds its ears detect. Which ones have meaning for it depends both on instinctive, inborn reactions and also on a certain amount of experience. Wild crows and herring gulls communicate each with their own kind by sounds that approximate a language. At Pennsylvania State University, Dr. Hubert Frings and his biologist wife have been discovering how much crows and gulls learn by listening to the calls of other birds. Crows in the United States, they find, have distinctive alarm notes inducing other crows to fly away, as well as distress calls when caught, and assembly calls given when they sight an owl or a cat. A recording of these calls on high-fidelity tape is sufficiently clear crow language to induce the same actions when played to wild crows in a woodland.

When these tape records are tested on crows in France, no response (or the wrong one) is seen. French crows assemble, rather than fly away, when they hear the alarm call of Pennsylvania crows. French herring gulls ignore completely the whole repertoire of signals vocalized by American herring gulls. The French birds don't seem to understand the foreign language.

Captive Pennsylvania crows, unable to travel and see the New World, do not respond normally to the calls of Maine crows. And conversely. But crows free to migrate between the two areas do come to understand both local dialects. There may even be some interchange between the birds of northern Europe and America, for the crows found in Maine during the winter react more to the calls of French crows than do crows summering in Maine. Crows wintering in Pennsylvania are more like Maine's summer birds in this respect. Migratory birds appear able to learn the meaning of calls from others of their own and even different kinds. Herein could be read a fine testimonial in favor of travel.

Smaller birds know one owl from another by its call, and will show this ability even toward imitations of owl notes made by man. Dr. Loye Miller of the University of California Museum in Berkeley discovered that small birds in the wild do not react, however, to the call notes of large owls. Bigger birds, which are endangered by large owls at one or another stage of life, do respond if the owl is of a kind native to the same area. None of these birds reacts to the calls of owls from distant regions. Nor do larger birds show awareness for the notes of small local owls that are unlikely to attack them.

All these revelations about language in ourselves and other animals make us wonder how early a parent and offspring begin communicating with each other. Certainly the mother crocodile hurries to the nest mound when she hears the cries of hatchlings far down in the debris and mud. She rips open the mound and lets out the youngsters. Does a human baby listen to its mother before birth? Recently, linguists have wondered about the lub-dupp, lub-dupp, lub-dupp from the mother's heartbeat. Primitive languages are full of repeat-syllabled words, comparable to familiar baby talk: da-da, ma-ma, gee-gee. Perhaps we are born with a strong preference for sounds in pairs, imitating the comforting sequence heard in the womb.

When you come to think about it, you realize that in most human societies a baby has a chance to listen to its mother's heart after birth too. She holds the child in her arms with its ear pressed against her chest, or she protects it under her blanket on her back, with its ear flattened against her skin between her shoulder blades. Surely the baby can hear as well as a doctor with a stethoscope cupped against these areas. We may yet discover an importance for a mother's heart sounds in the normal development of the child.

These days, all sorts of uses are being found for recorded sounds. The soft lub-dupp, lub-dupp of a relaxed mother's heartbeat was played recently over the loud-speaker system into a nursery room full of newborn babies. Outside the big picture window, a hospital technician with a clipboard kept a tally on the youngsters in the bassinets. Most of them soon went off to sleep. The rest appeared reasonably contented. The recording stopped. Within a few seconds a good many babies woke up; some began to cry. Then a new record was played: the rapid heartbeat from an excited woman. The sound was no louder, but all of the sleeping babies awoke immediately. Every infant grew tense, as though in fear. When the first recording was played again, peace spread through the nursery. Are its mother's heartbeat sounds a baby's first mood music?

Lub-dupp, lub-dupp, comes seventy times a minute from the heart at its normal pace, like a metronome of human life. For almost a century and a half, our old Terry mantel clock has been clucking out this soothing rhythm: tick-tock, tick-tock, marking the seconds. It is the tempo of a military band playing march music: oom-pah, oom-pah, left-right, left-right, with the bass drums and the brasses booming out the downbeat, the snare drums pulsing the up. With a downbeat each second—slightly slower than a human heart at rest—the cadence helps the squad march along indefinitely. Only on parade, for show and excitement, is the tempo increased to step the left foot forward seventy-two times a minute—just a little faster than the beat of a resting heart.

Our ears must be telling us something extremely fundamental when we are stirred by music, even though civilized man seems to have forgotten what it is. An inner response is waiting, just as instincts are, to be brought to the surface consciousness by thrilling rhythms. The English dramatist William Congreve described it simply in the late seventeenth century when he noted that "music hath charms..." Our great American essayist Paul Elmer More tried to be specific, and called it a "psychical storm, agitating to fathomless depths the mystery of the past within us."

Whatever it is, we should be grateful for possessing this rhythmic sense. Without it, the 23,500 vibration-sensitive cells in the inner ear might inform the brain only about noise, or warning sounds, or speech. Instead, these microscopic centers—each the size of a red blood cell—bestow upon us the bonus of music, of rhythm, and melody and harmony. They add extra dimensions to our lives.

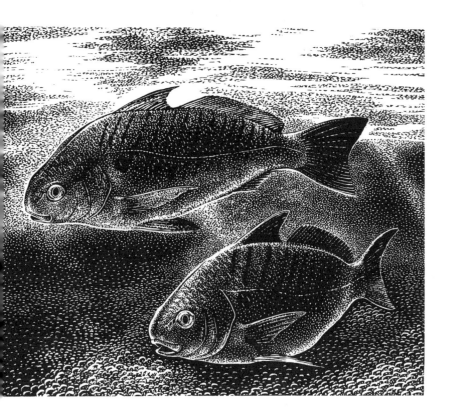

5. *The Noisy World of the Skin Diver*

NOT UNTIL after the first third of the twentieth century, when the human population of the continents had surpassed 200 million, did many people give much thought to the depths of the sea. It is almost as though they were pushed into it. Yet four-fifths of the world is covered by oceans. They form the largest, as well as the earliest, realm inhabited by living things. In ancient seas, countless eons ago, animals began making meaningful noises and detecting them. But whether crustaceans or fishes took the lead may never be known.

Even the existence of this animal communication by sound in the "silent world" of the oceans has been realized

49

widely by scientists only since the 1940's. Not until 1944 would our Navy Department bother to test an underwater communication system, although the one now in use was suggested seven years earlier than that by Dr. Maurice Ewing, the outstanding oceanographer who directs Columbia University's Lamont Geological Observatory. The very first explosion of a six-pound TNT depth charge at Dakar, West Africa, was detected with an underwater microphone ("hydrophone") some 3,100 miles away in the Bahamas. The vibrations crossed the width of the Atlantic Ocean in less than one hour. A test of this kind in 1960 reached the limit—halfway around the world from southwest of Australia to Bermuda in 223 minutes.

Underwater sounds went undetected for so long chiefly because of the barrier posed by the surface film. Vibrations in air are about 99.9 per cent reflected or absorbed as they strike a water surface. Vibrations within the water are imprisoned in the same way. Rarely can a skin diver hear underwater sounds past the air remaining in his ears.

Leonardo da Vinci is credited with recommending that a person listen to the handle of an oar dipped vertically into the water. Primitive fishermen in the South Seas and West Africa actually use this method, having invented it for themselves. Vibrations begun as underwater sounds are transmitted by the wood with enough energy for a human ear to notice if it is pressed against the handle. Fishermen who use this method rely upon the fact that fish are, as is now clear from scientific research, "incredibly garrulous."

Fishes were suspected of gossiping as far back as Aristotle's day. He observed some fish rubbing their gill arches together, and others shifting their internal organs in ways that seemed to produce vibrations in the swim bladder—a gas-filled bag lying in the body cavity just below the backbone and the kidneys. As far as he went, Aristotle was right.

The swim bladder does pick up and resonate, in this way amplifying all manner of vibrations in the body. A wide variety of fishes make special use of it, with definite drumming muscles extending from the backbone or the skull to the swim bladder. Contractions of these muscles throw the swim bladder into vibration, producing sounds transmitted to the surrounding water. Calls have this origin in drum fishes, sea perches, sea robins and gurnards, the "singing fish," and the lumpy toadfish. A similar technique allows the croaker and its kin to produce a roll of rapid grunts or croaks. Older and larger fishes pitch the note more than an octave below younger and smaller ones of the same kinds, showing that their voices change as they grow.

On the Yellow Sea and the China Sea, fishermen trying to sleep in their thin-hulled wooden ships have long complained that the chorus of croakers kept them awake. Along our own Atlantic shores in Chesapeake Bay, the normal influx of migrant croakers ready to spawn did keep sleepless a large number of Navy personnel and scientists during the spring and summer of 1942. A hydrophone network had been installed to warn coastal defenses if any Axis submarine approached. In late May the croaker invasion began, and during the evening hours the loudspeakers of the warning system sent out sounds resembling pneumatic drills breaking through concrete. At first no one could guess the cause, and many feared some new method of jamming was being tried out by the enemy already in our waters.

By the time the din had been traced to the croakers, the Bay held between 300 and 400 millions of these fish. Their average size had risen enough so that the loudest pitch came at middle C instead of nine notes higher. After July the swimmers departed again for the open Atlantic, and their return in later years was scarcely noticed because the coastal defense system had been equipped with croaker-proof filters which allowed the sound of submarine propellers to be heard.

Some noise-making fish reach the public ear in quite another guise. A popular ballad of a few years ago told of a homesick little Hawaiian who longed to return to his poi and his grass shack in Healakahua, where the humahumanukanuka apuaa went swimming by. A humahumanukanuka apuaa is a triggerfish which grunts in a rasping fashion, both when caught and while swimming in waters around our newest state. It is similar to the horse mackerel the ocean sunfish and the squirrelfish in that its sound comes from special teeth grated together in its throat.

The sea is full of sounds, for all manner of living things from shrimps to whales call back and forth. Men eavesdropping on the underwater world with the help of hydrophones have come up with every possible comparison: buzzing, cackling, chirping, clucking, crackling, croaking, drumming, grinding, groaning, grunting, moaning, snapping, squawking, squeaking, whining and whistling. In addition they have listed noises suggesting coal rattling down a chute, the dragging of heavy chains, a loose bearing on a reciprocating engine, the irregular put-put of an outboard motor about to stall, steaks sizzling, the dull roll of a soft-shoe dancer on the top of an empty barrel, and a band saw cutting through sheet metal.

Many of these sounds await identification, for it is one thing to hear and record them from a boat, and quite another to watch the animal in action. Some fish seem intent on remaining incognito, and become silent whenever they swim past a boat or through a light beam. Those in public aquaria grow loquacious, oblivious of their lack of privacy.

Records of sounds from captive fishes often match mystery calls heard from the open sea, revealing reliably which fish spoke out. Since 1946 a whole library of these sounds has been accumulating at the Narragansett Marine Laboratory of the University of Rhode Island, under the official title of "The Reference File of Biological Underwater Sounds." To give the public a chairside version, the Folkways Science Series recently released a long-playing record, one side with sounds heard in aquaria containing known kinds of fishes, and the other side the underwater sounds of biological origin taken in the Atlantic and Pacific oceans at depths from the surface to two thousand fathoms (a little over $2\frac{1}{4}$ miles down).

The host of unlike voices transform the sea into a party line from which each subscriber picks out his own messages. If François Rabelais could live again and hear them, he might wonder why four centuries elapsed without men of science giving attention to these sounds. His hero, Pantagruel, discoursed on the subject with the Skipper, and was told that the noises he heard at night from the sea were sounds from a battle the preceding winter, frozen solid in the air at that time and just now thawing out to become audible again. Calls from the true abysses do come from water close to the freezing point. But today's information groups them with sounds produced near the surface, all with a more believable origin.

In the dark depths there is a real need for sound to help potential mates find one another. Catfishes and others in the murky waters of shallow lakes and streams meet the same difficulty and solve it in the same way. The use of sound varies greatly, however, between the sexes. The male satinfin shiner defends a definite territory with thumping sounds while driving off another male. For a female he reserves his gentlest purring calls. Scientists have satisfied themselves by recording courtship sounds that the female usually needs to both hear and see her mate to be affected, or to sense him in some additional way—not just by a serenade alone. Apparently females do not like to be fooled. And the calls of the male can be useful even if they do not serve as a sure lure for the opposite sex. They clearly help him drive away other males who would compete for food needed by a mate and young.

Among the loudest calls recorded at the Narragansett Laboratory are those of the male toadfish in mating season, He roars like a foghorn, repeating the sound at thirty-second intervals. Later, while he guards the eggs he fathered, the sound emerges as a low, rough growl. A pet sea robin makes a purring sound when rubbed, but emits a burst of unpleasant noise when annoyed. When all alone, the sea robin often "talks" to itself.

Dr. Marie Poland Fish of the Narragansett Laboratory has learned to distinguish among fish calls showing "aggravation," "alarm" and "readiness for combat." The pitch of these sounds differs greatly, but most of the sound energy is in the vibration frequencies between 75 and 300 c.p.s. Dr. Fish noticed that among twenty-six different kinds of call makers only three raised their notes above 1,600 c.p.s. These stridulatory sounds went as high as 4,800 c.p.s.—almost four octaves above middle C. The "growl" of toadfishes off Bimini in the Bahamas, however, ranges as high as 6,000 c.p.s., which is really a shrill scream by human standards.

We can be sure that fishes hear the sounds we make, even though these aquatic creatures lack visible ears and are so like the water in sound-conducting characteristics that they are essentially transparent to sound vibrations. A fish hears perfectly, however, with only inner ears, close to the brain. Sounds from the water pass unhindered to these centers, and there are detected with a sensitivity comparable to man's best.

Inner ears are not the only organs of hearing for a fish. Dr. H. Kleerekoper and his associates at Canada's McMaster University have found other sound-sensitive centers in horned dace of Ontario streams. Horned dace (known also as creek chub) are most sensitive at 280 c.p.s., just above middle C. But they can be taught to respond to sounds over the whole range from 1 to 5,750 c.p.s. In the vicinity of 50 c.p.s., they can even distinguish between two notes as close together as one-fifth octave, which is better than some people can do. Above 2,000 and below 20,000 c.p.s., however, a vibration must be rich in energy for a horned dace to detect it.

With its inner ears removed surgically, a fish of this kind behaves normally and still responds to vibrations between 20 and 200 c.p.s., indicating that it has a standby hearing system. This remaining sensitivity to sound vibrations can be eliminated by cutting the nerve to the special sense organs of the lateral line on each side of the body. The fish remains "deaf" until the nerve regenerates, but never regains its ability to hear above 200 or below 20 c.p.s. in the ranges for which the inner ears are needed. Many other fishes likewise depend on the two sets of sense organs for hearing vibrations in the water about them. They rely on the lateral line organs for low pitches and the inner ears particularly for high.

A large number of different kinds of fishes are blind, but no fish is known to be naturally deaf. Those living in and around coral reefs must suffer at times from the din about them, for of underwater noises the most widespread and persistent by far comes from small animals of sea crannies. They are not fishes but shrimps, which rarely grow much beyond two inches in length. These noisiest neighbors in the world of the skin diver are called snapping shrimps or pistol shrimps because one claw is greatly enlarged and modified to form an effective water pistol. It is used in dueling, in repelling enemies and in capturing food. The combined efforts of millions of these animals just offshore has been credited with frightening pedestrians along the beaches of Japan. A single pistol shrimp in a jar of sea water can make a snap sharp enough to fracture the glass container. Yet no one is sure that the sound produced has any importance to the shrimps themselves.

In thinking about the sounds of underwater animals, we assume that they correspond closely to those with which we are familiar on land. Some sounds probably are incidental to other activities. Others are communication of a simple sort, alerting one member of a species to the presence and the direction of another. A few may convey extra meaning, such as alarm or discovery of food or readiness to mate. The earliest scientific report on fish sounds referred to one of these. It appeared in the 1905 *Proceedings* of the United States National Museum and has stood the test of time, although for almost 50 years few scientists would accept it as a true story. Theodore Gill had been studying the life history of sea horses. In one aquarium he had a male fish, in another a female. They could see each other through the glass, and their antics suggested recognition. One afternoon, Gill noticed that the male was making a series of sharp clicking sounds, each click loud enough to be heard through the room. Before long the female fish was responding, clicking in reply whenever the male called.

So simple are the sound messages conveyed by one animal to another of its kind that we accept animal conversations only in children's stories. We hesitate to credit any creature, particularly an aquatic one, with the ability to comment on man-made noises. Yet porpoises, which have warm blood, large brains and many special abilities, may prove capable of making far more meaningful sounds than any fish. Porpoises, or dolphins, which actually are toothed whales of small size, have been known to imitate human speech distinctly without encouragement. One at Marine Studios in Florida imitated a man's voice so well that his wife laughed heartily. Promptly the porpoise imitated her laughter! Perhaps when a playful porpoise nudges a person ashore from deep water, it is merely trying to clear the ocean of things that make strange sounds!

Dr. John C. Lilly, an experienced neurophysiologist, suspects that porpoises are unusually intelligent, as well as astonishingly cooperative in confinement. At a Communications Research Institute in the Virgin Islands, he is exploring the possibility of interspecies communication between man and dolphin. Whether the animals will prove able to learn a simple English more easily than Dr. Lilly and his associates can learn to bark, squawk, click, whistle, creak, blat and quack like porpoises, remains to be seen. If messages can get across, porpoises might even be induced to cooperate with fishermen, assisting workers in this ailing industry by finding, tracking, herding or even catching fish—in all of which activities porpoises are expert. These animals could help in many ways in man's exploration of the sea. But even more important than such assistance may be the fact that in man's own evolution he has now reached the point of attempting to communicate with nonhuman species.

Learning to identify and make use of underwater sounds is a new scientific game, a pioneer field just starting. It relies upon the same ability man has shown in recognizing birds and other land creatures by their calls. The challenge, however, is far greater. The denizens of the seas are infinitely varied and mysterious; most of them cannot be followed by any other method yet devised. Their voices, coming from the shallows and deeps, fairly cry for attention. Yet, though we listen and hold our breath to hear the better, we still have too little knowledge to identify many of the callers. Perhaps when listening to the sounds in the seas and fresh waters becomes as old as bird watching is today, the meaning of the calls and the individuality of the call makers will be recognized more fully. But at present few fields of outdoor inquiry offer more tantalizing experiences. It is as though the immensities of ocean were daring man to invade them, and to learn the secrets of the place whence he came so long ago.

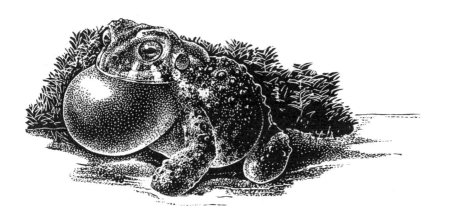

6. *The Sounds of the Seasons*

EACH TIME of year has its special meaning. As the seasons cycle past they offer repetitions of pleasures we have known: the welcome warmth of spring sunshine, the fragrances of summer flowers, the fruits of autumn, the lively flames of burning logs crackling in the fireplace on a winter night. We think of the world greening under April's showers, of July picnics, of October foliage and of the pure glistening whiteness of fresh snow reflecting a January sun.

The weather cannot tell us the time of year. It is too fickle. Any long record of daily temperatures for a single place contains a few winter days warm as cool spells in summer. During many autumns we could mistake a week or more for spring. We can, of course, match the calendar to the height of the sun in the sky at noon, or to the proportions of day and night. But with our eyes shut we can know the season far more delightfully by listening to the calls of animals around us.

Summer is not swallow time, for swallows arrive in the spring—all of them. Summer is the season when the nights are full of chirping crickets and the long twilights ring with the *peent* of nighthawks overhead. It means for us the bang

57

of heavy-bodied chafers against the window screens, and the never-ending call of the whippoorwill. Summer days have come with the intense whine of a cicada, or a field full of grasshoppers leaping and snapping their wings.

The elk bugle in the autumn. Moose bellow and rattle their fully-spread racks of antlers against low branches of alders in the swales. Autumn is katydid time: katydids in the trees; katydids on the sprays of goldenrod flowers when the night is too dark to see the color. From grass-blades and shrubbery all day long, green grasshoppers with tremendous antennae zip out distinctive calls, making the most of the last warmth from the sun before frost turns the final page of their music.

And winter? It's the cheery calls of chickadees hunting for seeds wherever they can be found, and for insects dormant in the bark. It's the yank-yank note of nuthatches ignoring gravity on tree trunks. It's the silence of nights in which the occasional hoot of an owl, the crunch of snow under the feet of a deer or hare and the pistol crack of ice on the river all stand out in sharp contrast, with few leaves to block the spread of sound.

Regardless of the calendar and thermometer, winter is gone when a northbound wedge of geese honks from the sky and peepers chorus along the streams. Buds will burst for sure in the week when we hear the first mating calls of frogs and toads in the night air, and the exuberant songs of migrant birds by day.

Season after season we listen for our friends to call, to remind us how reliably living things continue in a pattern established long before man was here to notice. Often the voice is as distinctive as the form of the creature. We wonder what the season was when the first land animal made a deliberate sound. What creatures were there to hear it?

Today we can find a faint repetition of this earliest note when we overturn a stone or log in the warmer parts of our country and disturb a scorpion. Scorpions appeared in the world of Devonian times, four hundred million years ago, as perhaps the earliest land animals able to give an audible warning. The modern scorpion reacts to the rush of air as we lift its roof. It raises pincer-tipped claws, so suggestive of those a New England lobster carries. The scorpion arches its tail, bringing the tip above its back, the sharp stinger on the end ready with venom in case we come too close. As the tail rises we hear the squeak, as though the joints were rusty. This slight noise accompanies the same threatening gesture in scorpions all over the world. It is produced by the rubbing together of special rough surfaces on the body. What season was it when the first scorpion squeaked?

Everywhere, the songs of insects are far more familiar than the scraping notes of scorpions. These obvious calls date back only about three hundred million years, to the time when modern coal was the wood of living trees. Most insect sounds are a prerogative of the males, a near-monopoly that has stood the test of time. Male crickets chirped and male grasshoppers fiddled through the heyday and downfall of the dinosaurs. Their calls outlasted the Ice Ages, and seem likely to continue every summer as long as the earth is habitable by any living thing.

Just as bird calls are distinctive and serve in proclaiming possession of territory, so also each insect musician plays his specific tune. Others of his kind recognize it. So can we, if our ears are sharp. With our words katydid and cricket—from the Old French *criquet* ("creak-ay")—we try to capture the identifying rhythms. Just before the turn of the century, the eminent naturalist Samuel H. Scudder attempted to write in musical form the calls of the grasshoppers and crickets he knew so well around his New England home. Today his notes seem crude by comparison with modern high-fidelity recordings and the analyses made possible with electronic instruments.

Our own preference has been for the camera and flashgun. A tree cricket shrilling softly at three in the morning has been irresistible to us, its call like the ringing of elfin bells. The note continues while the pastel green insect stands with its wings quivering at right angles to its back, held up in a way that provides extra resonance for the sound.

Tree crickets, like katydids and long-horned grasshoppers, make their sounds by rubbing together a scraper on one wing cover near its base and a series of ridges or pegs on the other, like stroking a file or a comb quickly with a fingernail. These insects are connoisseurs of pitch and rhythm, and listen intently to sounds in the surrounding shrubbery with delicate ears set in their front legs just below the joint corresponding to the knee. A single male can produce as a sort of monologue the calls we imitate by "Katy," "Katy Did" and "Katy Didn't," with two, three or four strokes of the file and scraper in quick succession. Katydids and long-horned grasshoppers give their distinctive theme songs with a brief, quivering shrug, raising only the base of the wing covers and seldom drawing attention to themselves as they stand, green as the foliage, listening for a reply.

The strength of the call from a katydid or a cricket is a good measure of the insect's readiness to mate. When other males sense its power, they keep their distance in proportion, leaving the largest territory to the loudest singer. Usually the call vanishes after mating and shows that the male temporarily is bowing out of the contest for a spouse. In some long-horned grasshoppers this seems highly logical, for the male may decrease in body weight by as much as 40 per cent when he transfers to the female his large sac of sperm cells. In a few days, as he recovers his weight and sexual readiness, his call returns too. Appropriately enough, the females are impressed by vigor and ordinarily choose the male with the loudest song.

A clue to the manner of call making and hearing can be found in the length of the antennae of crickets, katydids and grasshoppers, although these "feelers" have nothing to do with sound. Crickets and katydids are "long horns." Short-horned grasshoppers are the familiar insects—the locusts—that crackle and splutter like burning underbrush when the summer sun has parched the fields and people hunt for shade in which to open their picnic baskets. Locusts watch alertly while clinging to a tall stem or standing on the ground, drawing attention by sounding off. Many of them leap into the air and circle like helicopters, snapping out their calls from a few feet above the ground before settling on a bit of bare earth as though it were a landing field or parade ground. In almost all cases their sounds are made by rough areas on the thighs of the rear pair of legs rubbing against the outer surface of the wing covers. Some grasshoppers have a file on the wing and a scraper on the thigh. Others have these stridulatory surfaces disposed in exactly the opposite way. Females, too, may call softly. Both sexes hear the sound through ears on each side, close to the region where the rear legs arise from the body.

Courting locusts are in no hurry as they follow through the age-old sequence of instinctive motions. It takes patience to recognize when a male's snapping self-advertisement changes to a sort of "general song" as he sights another insect of the right size and shape. The "reply song" of the unmated female is softer, and leads to a duet during which the locusts of unlike sex approach each other. The final number is as short as a brilliant encore. It is the "courtship song," so highly characteristic of each species that there is almost no chance for unlike kinds of insects to mate and give rise to defective hybrids. For maintaining the reproductive purity of each race, these love songs are highly important.

Eye-minded man cannot help but wonder at species segregated by their sounds. Only by reminding ourselves of the differences in dimensions between their lives and ours can we appreciate fully their reliance upon a seasonal display of coded calls. How else could a small animal efficiently stake a claim to a bush or a clump of grass, and with the same gesture invite an unseen mate to approach? Usually the insect has no time to waste, for a single season encompasses its entire period of maturity. A week or two (or perhaps a month) affords all the chances to reproduce its kind it will ever have. Any individual reaching adulthood early or late is almost certain to leave no offspring. Once this urgency is realized, the furious fiddling of the crickets and their kin becomes understandable.

Perhaps we should be more surprised that so many of these insect musicians are shy enough to stop in the middle of a note if disturbed in any way. Crickets and katydids and grasshoppers all make their calls loudly, as public pronouncements, only when the world seems ready to listen. How different these insects are from the cicadas, which will buzz vigorously when picked up, and shrill an even louder protest when approached by their mortal enemies, the cicada-killer wasps! Yet the cicadas have a still smaller proportion of their total life span in which to start another generation on its way. Some of them spend as many as seventeen silent years developing to maturity, and then a few weeks at most before death ends the loud courtship song.

Cicadas are also called "locusts" and "harvest flies." Their song comes from unique drumlike tymbals, one on each side of the sturdy body halfway back from the head. There air-filled cavities serve as resonators whenever special muscles set the drum membranes vibrating. These insects send out an intense siren whine on hot summer days in temperate lands, and even noisier calls at sunrise and sunset hours in a tropical jungle. Some of them sound like mechanical toys whose whirring clockwork slows almost to a stop, only to pick up sharply, run down again, and finally cease altogether. So insistent is the note that it is often easy to find the male where he clings to the bark of a tree, inviting mates to come from any side. These insects have no obvious ears, but clearly hear the sounds we do. Females heed the invitation, and dart at high speed through the woodland to settle beside the singers.

When we refer to the calls of insects as love songs or invitations or signs of resentment, we are speculating without admitting it. It is like sweeping dust behind the door. As we try to interpret the sounds of animals at various times of year, almost certainly we find importance in some that have no meaning for the animals themselves. By association only do we gain pleasure in distinguishing between the soft hum of a hawk moth's wings as it hovers before a bloom in the dusk and the more vigorous whirr of a hummingbird visiting the same flower at dawn. These are incidental sounds of summer, when moth or bird and blossom coincide.

We've wondered, when visiting tropical America where it is summer all the time, whether the "clicker butterflies" (*Ageronia*) find meaning in the sounds they make. These insects rest head downward on the trunks of trees, silently waving their wings as though to display the bright pastel spots. Every few minutes a male darts into the air, snaps his wings audibly, just as though clicking his heels. Then he returns to the bark perch for a pirouette or two. His flight is clearly a courtship gesture. But does the sound, which suggests the snap of human fingers, attract a mate? Perhaps it is no more than the butterfly equivalent of the slapping together of a pigeon's wings when the bird first rises into the air. While in Brazil, Charles Darwin noticed these insects as a pair were chasing each other. He "distinctly heard a clicking noise, similar to that produced by a toothed wheel passing under a spring catch. The noise was continued at short intervals, and could be distinguished at about twenty yards' distance."

Even when a sound is incidental to the summer activities of an animal, it can serve a purpose. The whine of a mosquito comes from the rapid movement of its wings in flight. We know it too well, and cringe when we hear it, expecting to be bitten. Male mosquitoes are attuned to this sound, detecting it by means of specially sensitive regions of the antennae. Long hairs there vibrate in unison with the wing sound of the correct species of female. Male yellow-fever mosquitoes are attracted most strongly by vibrations of 500 to 550 per second; their mates produce the appropriate sound with wings beating at rates of 449 to 603. Even in the presence of loud background noises, the males locate them. Sometimes, however, they are fooled and come in countless hordes to electric power stations that whine at the proper pitch. Millions may be found in a heap at the bottom of the cooling fins on a big transformer. They have cooked themselves by alighting momentarily upon its hot vibrating surface.

The most terrifying of all insect flight sounds is met during a seasonal visit by migratory grasshoppers, such as those of the Near East and many parts of Africa. They were the "eighth plague" to afflict the Egyptians during Moses' day. Darwin quoted *Revelation* for those he encountered on the plains of Patagonia: "And the sound of their wings was as the sound of chariots of many horses running to battle." Then he added, "Or rather . . . like a strong breeze passing through the rigging of a ship." In level flight these insects make relatively little sound we can hear. But when a cloud-sized swarm lands or takes off, the vibrations are almost deafening. We heard them clearly in Africa despite the engine noise of the light airplane in which we were flying, and saw the locusts rise at midmorning from the ruined croplands as though the tan soil itself had acquired wings.

Apparently the flight sounds of these grasshoppers—chiefly in the range between seventeen and twenty vibrations per second—are important to the insects themselves. Deafened locusts show little interest in taking off with the rest of the population. But a whole mass of intact grasshoppers will leave the ground if they hear a recording of flight noises played to them. Whether they can be kept flying to exhaustion and death by this means, as Chinese city dwellers claim to have done with English sparrows ("rice birds") alarmed by the din of gongs and firecrackers, is a question to which the International Locust Control Commission is seeking an answer.

It was wing vibrations that William Butler Yeats celebrated when he wrote of the "bee-loud glade." His ears delighted in the sound, as have so many others before and since Yeats's time. Most of us recognize the slight variations in tone as the nectar gatherer forages from one flower to another. It makes a quiet, low-pitched sound, quite different from the snarling whine of the same insects when they are seriously disturbed. Their sound changes too, during the normal growth of a colony, as it prepares to swarm. In 1959 an electronic engineer described a monitoring device he had used, attached to a beehive. Whenever the sounds from within took on the preswarming pitch, a microphone and amplifier system picked up the vibrations, identified them automatically, and sent a warning to the beekeeper in his home.

Honeybees are attentive to flight sounds too. At the entrance to the hive, the workers who serve as guard bees pay no attention to other workers about to alight. They do seem sensitive to the pitch of the wing beat from robber bees while these are still some distance off. Similarly, while watching the honeybees coming to flowers in summertime, anyone can notice the difference when a bee-sized, bee-shaped, bee-colored dronefly arrives. Despite its striking similarities, even in behavior, the mimicking fly gives away its deception by its sound. Yet some mimics imitate even in this. Recently a case of "audio mimicry" was found, in

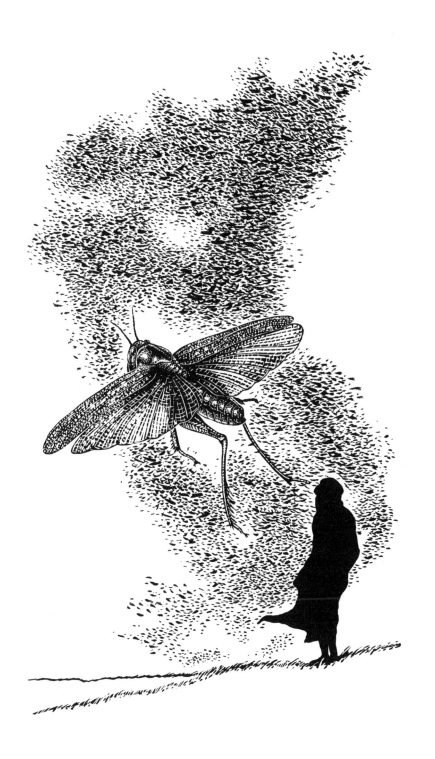

which a fly uses a wingbeat rate of 147 strokes per second while hovering near the wasps it resembles. The particular wasp flies with 150 wing strokes per second and, to people with normal hearing, the two flight sounds are indistinguishable. Presumably, fly-catching birds are deceived and avoid the mimicking flies.

One season after another for an immensity of time, the sounds of insects remained the most distinctive animal noises on earth. Only about 150 million years ago were they joined by the cries of creatures whose bodies provided "tongue and lung," the features Aristotle recognized as the requirements for a voice. It was almost as though the insects of many thousand kinds were so many pied pipers leading the animals with backbones out of the seas and the streams and the swamps, into the air and over the land to the homes they occupy today. Birds and furry mammals appeared, chirping and yelping in pursuit of insects. Frogs and toads joined the chorus every spring, continuing to the present on an insect diet.

The emergence from the waters is re-enacted every year. Amphibians put aside their silent tadpole days, grow legs and absorb the swimming tail. Always they return, however, to the ponds and marsh margins for a springtime choral symphony that has a strong aesthetic appeal for man. Many a neighbor who would not admit to being a naturalist thrills to the peeping of the tiny frogs with big voices soon after the disappearance of the winter snow and ice. The water may be barely above the freezing point, yet the peepers are calling for mates and starting a new generation on its aquatic, vegetarian, tadpole way.

These nightly serenades tell us of spring, that skunk cabbages have opened their strange flowers to early insects in the swamp, that pollen-filled catkins are swinging "like laden censers" on birch and alder, that bloodroot will soon unfold its cloaklike leaves and raise nodding buds of snowy white into open-petaled flowers.

Fresh foliage of countless hues spreads to the light as warty toads add their trilling voices to the peepers' concert. Later in the season come the explosive notes of slippery-skinned frogs. Last of all is the deeply resonant *ronk . . . ronk . . . ronk* of big bullfrogs patronizing permanent ponds in which their young can achieve a length of four inches or more before transforming into insect-catching bassos of the land.

In the tropics, where spring rains fall in every month, the chorusing of amphibians is part of the night—every night. People who live there continue to enjoy the calls and, in several islands of the West Indies, have increased their pleasure by introducing foreign talent. On Jamaica we met the "whistling frog" of Martinique, brought to the British island from the French one by Lady Blake, the wife of Jamaica's former governor. She became so enchanted by the double-note call of this little tree frog that she arranged for some of the singers to be released around Government House on the Liguanea Plains. Now the whistler has spread into the nearby campus of the University College of the West Indies and made itself at home. Its scientific name, *Eleutherodactylus martinicensis*, is twice as long as its body, and visitors who look for the vocalist seldom believe that this midget can be the one with the loud call. Children showed us where the whistlers spend the day in the metal boxes protecting water meters, in the lawn in front of homes, and helped us catch a few to watch in the evening. After dark each frog's gray throat swells at intervals with air, readying the vocal mechanism for the powerful "Bo-PEEP."

By choosing the season in the Temperate Zone, these pleasures can be found close by. Anywhere in New England during a summer evening, a note suggesting a bird's chirp is likely to be the short loud trill of the gray tree frog, a two-inch relative of the spring peepers. It repeats the call at intervals of many seconds, giving anyone with a flashlight a sporting chance to find the amphibian clinging inconspicuously to the side of a tree, showing his lemon-yellow throat during the instant of trilling.

The southeastern states are home to the barking tree frog, of slightly larger size. From high in the forest it sends out a series of nine or ten raucous syllables. But in spring and summer, after rains, it descends to water level and there produces single explosive notes. These breeding choruses of barking tree frogs are grouped into trios like barbershop harmonizers, each individual singing a different note. Members of a trio recognize a leader and follow a regular "peep order," with one frog always the first to cry *toonk*, and another invariably waiting to be last in sequence.

Toads and frogs have eardrums set flush with the sides of the head, and show special awareness for the sounds of their own kinds. Rarely does a hybrid appear through the crossing of unlike species breeding in the same pond. Hybrids, however, can be produced in the laboratory. Their voices are intermediate between the two parental types, showing that the songs are inborn and not learned.

Amphibians pay attention to many sounds from the world around them, not just to mating calls. A rustling in the bushes is enough to stop a chorus, to begin a long period of complete silence. Or the shriek of one frog seized by a snake will send every other frog on a reckless leap for the water, where the animals dive and hide themselves among the bottom plants. Where frog-catching snakes are numerous, even the vibration of human footsteps through the earth may be enough to induce a whole series of shrieks and leaps. Half an hour of quiet waiting may pass before a few daring frogs break the spell, sending out tentative notes as though to test whether the danger has gone away.

It seems unlikely that the snake that stalks a frog or, for that matter, an insect or a mouse, hears any calls these potential victims make. Snakes lack external ears, and presumably cannot hear one another hiss. Even the warning rattle of the rattlesnakes seems to be a threatening sound important only to other creatures. Yet the whole body of a snake serves it as an ear, sensitive to vibrations in the ground. So well do most snakes detect the approach of footsteps, whether of man or of grazing cow, that the reptile slithers off and avoids being discovered.

We who live in the North Temperate Zone seldom realize our good fortune in the variety of animal calls enlivening our shores and fields and woodlands. In addition to the seasonal stridulations of insects and the voicing of amphibians, we enjoy more variety of complex bird songs than are to be heard anywhere else on earth. The thrushes and orioles may spend the winter in the tropics or the Southern Hemisphere, as do so many other birds. But they are almost silent there. Only north of the Torrid Zone do they court their mates and raise their young, defending territory with songs of great distinction.

Bird voices can utter as many as four different notes simultaneously, and produce a rapid sequence of separate sounds faster than any human ear can follow. By use of tape recorders it is now possible to play back bird calls slowed to a quarter or an eighth of their normal speed, and to marvel at the performance. The winter wren sings 130 notes in a song lasting just over seven seconds, repeating this performance endlessly with almost no variations. The wood thrush provides innovations in its three-part song, and ranges widely and rapidly through pitches from 1,640 to 8,900 vibrations per second. One individual wood thrush, from which fifty-five songs were recorded, did not repeat itself a single time. The ever-fresh melody combined two variants in the first part of the song, five versions of the second part, and nine of the third part. Some of the notes were slurred smoothly over nearly an octave within a two-hundredth of a second.

Thrushes, which frequent woodland borders all over the world, are quite justifiably the most famous singers among wild birds. Usually they slip inconspicuously through the undergrowth, blending with the patterns of fallen leaves. If it were not for their voices, they would almost surely be overlooked by most people. Actually it is the song that is famous, rather than the bird. From Keats's extravagant ode to the nightingale no one can learn that the singer is a slender brown bird with a reddish tail, the European counterpart of the American hermit thrush. Nor has any impartial jury yet decided whether the nightingale, the hermit thrush or the chama thrush of India (where it earns a similarly high regard) is the most accomplished singer of all. Perhaps this is because the voices of these birds are best appreciated only in their native woodlands, which are so far apart.

Most of the notes in bird songs arise from a special syrinx deep in the chest region, remote from the equivalent of our voice box (larynx) and served by muscles which regulate pitch and tone quality. No one quite understands how this complex musical device operates, although its structure correlates with the songs produced. Among sparrowlike birds alone, five different forms of the syrinx have been recognized, based upon the number and arrangement of the muscles and the vibrating membranes.

Despite this great variety of calls available to birds, our feathered friends produce additional sounds important to them in communication. The drumming of a grouse standing on a hollow log in spring is the beat of wings, at close to forty strokes per second. The tapping of a woodpecker on a dead stub or a tin roof requires an especially sturdy beak and a brain that is almost immune to jarring shock. Yet these sounds are distinctive to our ears and to those of the birds themselves.

The red-headed woodpecker and the red-bellied woodpecker engage in mutual tapping. A male bird will call from his roost hole at dawn, and his mate fly to him from where she perched through the dark hours. She alights near the doorway and hears him tapping inside the tree hole. She joins in the noisemaking from outside. Dr. Lawrence Kilham, who has watched these birds for years near Washington, D. C., believes that the mutual tapping serves to strengthen the mating bond between the two birds, and perhaps indicates agreement on the site chosen for the nest hole.

Listening to the sounds of animals around us in every season, we learn more of individual lives. We come to recognize a message in a dog's bark or a robin's warning churk of "Cat!" Yet the world of each creature is as different from ours as its calls. Our most critical observation is needed to avoid crediting human motives and appreciation to non-human kinds of life. Some songs of birds represent exuberance, a spending of energy without other significance. But we should not forget that the sounds of animals form a code, often hidden in a wealth of confusing details. Each animal has its own code book, its own scale of values. In the range of sounds to which it is sensitive, it picks out only those syllables with special meaning. In seeking to break the code we must identify these syllables and learn their significance to the animal itself. Only then will the creature's actually simple language become one that man can understand.

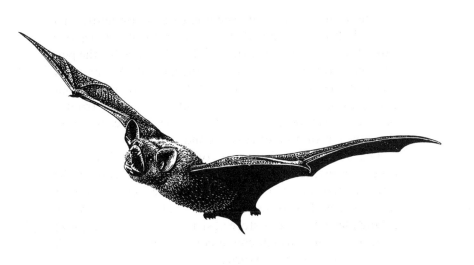

7. *Echoes of Importance*

ONE OF our most cherished abilities is our skill in recognizing the directions from which sounds come. Even without using our eyes, our hearing allows us to construct a mental picture of our surroundings and to be aware of changes as they occur. Sound actually affords some advantages over light in helping us keep apprised of life near by. Sound travels around corners and tells us of events that are out of sight. From large surfaces it echoes back to our ears and, unconsciously, our brains use this information too.

Our auditory direction sense makes us a fair target for commercial campaigns to promote stereophonic music, aimed at selling additional equipment said to bring a three-dimensional orchestra into a private living room. But our ears are far too sensitive for the illusion to be perfect unless we are willing to listen through earphones, with our heads in a fixed position. The illusion is tarnished if we so much as turn our heads, for the orchestra we hear seems to shift and remain straight ahead of our nose.

One of the pleasures in listening to a live orchestra in a music hall is in facing whichever instrument catches our attention. We turn to the right end of the stage for the percussion section and to the left for the harpist. We savor, as we turn, the slight differences in the sound pattern our ears pick up. We turn, in fact, until the sound from a particular part of the orchestra reaches both ears within the same ten-thousandth of a second.

The astonishing feature of our ability to detect any difference greater than a ten-thousandth of a second in the time of arrival of a sound, earlier at one ear and later at the other, is that we use it without realizing just what is taking place. In a clock store at striking time, we recognize "automatically" which chime comes from each clock. A blindfolded man, free to turn as he wishes at the center of a circle fifty feet across, can point accurately to whichever musician plays a sustained note, among eighteen instrumentalists spaced equally around the circle.

For the ears and brain working together to detect delays exceeding a ten-thousandth of a second is truly remarkable. Olympic sporting events are measured only to the nearest tenth of a second, and horse races to the nearest fifth. Yet there is no question in our minds whenever sound reaches one ear appreciably before the other. The greatest difference possible, in fact, is ten ten-thousandths of a second, which occurs whenever a noise comes over a shoulder from extreme right or left. The sound needs ten ten-thousandths of a second to travel the eight inches around the head after reaching the first ear before it strikes the other.

In striving for the illusion of a live orchestra along one wall of our living rooms, the acoustic engineers place their sensitive microphones one on each side of the music-hall stage. Notes from the piano and the harp reach the left microphone significantly before they do the right one. Sounds from the percussion section are picked up in the reverse order. When the two microphones are linked through separate circuits to the speakers in our homes, we hear a plucked chord on the harp through the left speaker before we do through the right. Our ears tell us that the harp is to the left. But we cannot eliminate the difference in time of sound arrival at our two ears by facing the left speaker.

Engineers cannot eliminate the echoes and reverberations of the music from walls and furnishings in our homes, although our ears detect them and tell us plainly that we are in no music hall. The best the stereophonic equipment can do is to transport our living rooms to the middle of the music hall, and let us hear the orchestra on the stage through two or more small portholes in the living-room wall—the portholes being the speakers at left and right. This is completely different from the thrilling illusion possible in our homes by listening through earphones when the pickup microphones in the music hall are the distance apart of the two ears on a human head. Yet no practicable compromise has yet been found.

The one real gain from all the attempts to let us hear music with a sense of "presence" is a fuller realization of how remarkably sensitive we are to differences in what our two ears hear, and our readiness to interpret echoes. Even blind men, who rely so heavily upon their other senses in avoiding obstacles, rarely realize how much their learned abilities depend upon hearing. Often they believe they are sensing objects ahead through the pores in their skin. Yet if their ears are plugged, the so-called "facial vision," which many sightless people claim, vanishes completely.

Echoes of which most people are aware come through the open windows of an automobile as it proceeds along a highway at a steady rate. The sound is chiefly "white noise" of mixed vibration frequencies arising from the motor and tires plus vibrations of the body, reflected from obstacles along the route. It is a hiss, a steady one as the car goes through a tunnel, or coming in regular blips from concrete guardrail posts, or somewhat more prolonged opposite each parked auto we pass along the roadside. With our eyes closed and a little practice in listening to these echoes, we can know our position remarkably well along a regularly traveled route. The differences allow us to distinguish among a parked large car, a compact or foreign model, a motorcycle, and a pedestrian waiting to cross. The pedestrian sounds "bigger" if his arms are full of parcels reflecting the sound. Yet none of these echoes reaches our ears for more than a moment.

With no special training we can do even more while blindfolded but with ears exposed. If we hold between thumb and forefinger a metal "cricket" such as some lecturers use in signaling for the next slide, and cup the other hand around it in the form of a shield directing the clicks away from us, our ears are protected from the sharp sound itself and we can hear its echo returning from buildings. By using such a noisemaker in a small parabolic horn, a person can detect trees six inches in diameter at a distance of several feet. These feats are simple versions of what sightless people accomplish by listening to the echoes of their footsteps or tapping cane, and of the way a flying bat can dodge wire obstacles as fine as a human hair or chase tiny insects as prey in the night.

In a forest of small trees, a shout is echoed back from many trunks. We rarely hear the echoes, however, because the ear ignores them. By using a tape recorder, it is possible to play back the record in the reverse sequence—echoes first and then the shout. The echoes become obvious and also clearly higher in pitch than the shout itself. This is because high-pitched sounds reflect as good echoes from small trees, whereas low-pitched sounds reverberate and are scattered in all directions. The echo of a "white noise" from small obstacles in its path is high pitched for the same reason that the sky is blue. White light from the sun includes a mixture of low-frequency vibrations (red) and high frequencies (blue). Molecules of air scatter its low frequencies and reflect to our eyes principally the remainder—the blue. If we heard the echoes of white noises more regularly, we would probably call them "blue noises" too.

One of the essential features of all vibrations, whether of ocean waves, sound waves, radio waves or light waves, is that the higher the frequency of waves per second, the shorter each wave must be. The higher the pitch of a note rises and the greater its vibration rate, the shorter its wave length becomes. Yet to send back a good echo, an obstacle needs to be two or three times as broad as the wave that strikes it is long. This is sometimes evident along a sea coast, where water waves pass a slender spar or buoy without commotion, only to be reflected by a long jetty.

If we want to bounce sound waves from small obstacles and listen to the echoes as a means for learning the direction and distance to the obstacle, we need to use the shortest waves possible, and hence the highest pitch of sound. Bats discovered these advantages in high-pitched sounds more than fifty million years ago. Man took until the late 1930's to apply the same techniques in his military installations of sonar ("SOund Navigation And Ranging").

Sound waves, of course, are much shorter than ocean waves. A middle-C tone of 256 vibrations per second has a wave length of 51 inches, and only a reflecting surface as big as a billboard will give a clear echo. The high notes from a metal cricket are probably close to five octaves above middle C, with waves about $1\frac{1}{2}$ inches long suitable for echoing from trees six inches in diameter. The cry of a bat, inaudible to our ears because its pitch is so high, includes frequencies up to 130,000 vibrations per second, with wave lengths down to 1/10 of an inch. Its small mouth can concentrate these short sound waves effectively and its ears pick up the echoes from obstacles ahead.

Bats are so much creatures of the fading twilight and night hours, and so many of them fly high above the ground, that they escape notice. Yet of all the many types of furry mammals, bats outnumber in kinds and as individuals all except the gnawing rodents. In the temperate zones they specialize as insect catchers, taking victims in mid flight or hovering in front of foliage and picking up insects from the surface. Tropical bats include many with these habits, as well as fruit-eating and nectar-sipping bats, fish-catching bats and, in the New World, the blood-lapping vampires.

With one exception, all of the large fruit-eating bats need vision in finding their way about. They are helpless if blindfolded. The exception (*Rousettus*, found from Burma to equatorial Africa) will use its eyes if it has enough light to see by, but can navigate by ear, listening to the echoes of clicking sounds made with its tongue. These clicks escape through the open corners of its mouth as higher-pitched equivalents of those we can produce by repeated sucking-and-tongue movements such as are often used to indicate disapproval ("tsk-tsk"). *Rousettus*' calls and excellence of hearing allow it to dodge vertical wires as small as 1/25 of an inch in diameter.

Without exception, the smaller bats behave as though they were blind. They manage spectacularly well in complete darkness so long as their hearing is intact, and could be said to "see with their ears." Among their number are some that click so softly as to be called "whispering bats." Others scan their surroundings with high-frequency sounds of a single pitch. Still others, including the familiar insectivorous bats of temperate America, employ loud ultrasonic cries which drop in pitch as much as an octave within a five-hundredth of a second—a regular variation which justly earns them the name of "frequency-modulation bats" (FM bats).

"Whispering bats" feed mostly upon tropical fruits, but take insects found resting on the vegetation. Apparently they never chase insects on the wing, and are masters of hovering. Their calls consist of extremely brief clicks so faint that only the very best microphones and sound-detecting equipment are affected by them. Rarely do they make any noise audible to man's ears. Many of their cries range as high as 150,000 vibrations per second.

The famous vampire is a medium-sized bat with the whispering habit. It hovers over a sleeping horse or man, then reaches out with razor-sharp teeth to cut through the skin and induce the blood to flow freely. A vampire takes the warm blood as delicately as a cat laps milk. Dogs, however, are rarely bitten by these bats, which may indicate that a dog's hearing is acute enough at the high pitches a vampire uses for echolocating its large victims that the dog awakens and frightens away the bat. Dr. Donald R. Griffin, professor of zoology at Harvard University and foremost authority on bat calls, has suggested that "hearing ear" dogs might be trained to warn of a vampire's approach, compensating for man's deafness in the ultrasonic range somewhat as "seeing eye" dogs aid the blind. Since vampires often carry rabies to their victims, the idea has another practical side.

The bats used by artists as models for illustrations intended to terrify people are usually the harmless horseshoe bats of Europe, Asia, Africa and Australia. These insect catchers have a double fold of membranes around the nose and mouth. This is the "horseshoe" which serves as a horn concentrating the high-frequency calls into a narrow beam of sound which can be swept back and forth as one might turn a flashlight. These bats scan their surroundings, and seem particularly well equipped for doing so even while resting downward from some support. Their hip joints are extraordinarily flexible, permitting the bat to swivel itself through almost a complete circle while scanning for an insect victim. When the sound reflects from a gnat or beetle, the bat darts out and captures a meal. As the British zoologist J. D. Pye pointed out, a bat is "a highly successful self-directed missile that relies on its targets for fuel."

The chirps of a horseshoe bat last from a twentieth to a tenth of a second, which is very long for a call used in echolocating food. Apparently the bat's ears can make use of an echo even while the animal's mouth and vocal cords are engaged in producing the cry. Seemingly, too, a horseshoe bat recognizes whether an insect victim is flying toward it or away, and adjusts its pursuit tactics accordingly. This extra ability may even simplify our understanding of bat uses for sound, since it corresponds to an experience to which we are all accustomed.

Whenever we ride a train we realize that its whistle or klaxon horn produces one constant pitch of note. Yet, as a blaring locomotive passes us at a station platform, the pitch of its whistle or horn drops sharply at the instant of passage. Known as the Doppler effect after its discoverer, this change is due to the movement of the train toward us and then away again. As the locomotive approaches, its whistle produces sound waves which are compressed by the train's own speed, shortening the wave length and raising the pitch for anyone on the ground ahead. As the train sweeps away again, the sound waves from the whistle traveling back to people on the station platform behind are drawn out by the locomotive's speed, lengthening each wave and lowering its pitch. Correspondingly, the echo of an insect flying away from a horseshoe bat would come back to the bat's ears as a lower pitch than the cry itself, whereas one from an approaching insect would be in a higher key. Surely a bat able to use any echo while the call is still issuing from its throat could learn even more from an echo with a slightly different pitch.

The common insectivorous bats of North America and Europe are FM bats, each of whose loud, high-pitched calls lasts but a few thousandths of a second. During that time the pitch is modulated smoothly. The abundant little brown bat begins each chirp at about ninety thousand vibrations per second, and sweeps it downward in pitch to end at forty-five thousand. A cry of this kind contains only about fifty sound waves altogether, with no two of them in the same key.

Ordinarily, an FM bat repeats its call ten to twenty times a second as it flies along. When it detects an interesting echo, however, it steps up the rate to as many as two hundred chirps per second, decreasing the length of each cry to about one thousandth of a second. Often the vibration rate rises slightly as though in excitement, without losing the FM characteristic. In describing these changes for a red bat responding to tossed pebbles or to wads of wet cotton batting fired from a pea shooter, Dr. Griffin translated the calls as "putt . . . . . putt . . . . put . . . pit . . pit . . pit pit pit pit-pit-pit-bizzz," with the bat brain interpreting the echoes in true fighter-pilot jargon: "June bug at two o'clock."

Of the group with frequency-modulated cries, the fish-catching bats are especially intriguing. However, no one is yet sure how well they can detect minnows through the water surface and echolocate a victim. The best known (*Noctilio*, a denizen of northern South America and northward into Mexico) uses the sharp gafflike hooks on its hind claws in plucking minnows out of their element. *Noctilio* has co-operated by fishing from a pan seventy-eight inches by thirty inches and two inches deep, flying skillfully to do so over the floor of a screened porch only eight feet wide. The bat's wing span is about twenty inches, and its fishing succeeded far oftener than chance alone would explain.

Noctilio has been called the "harelipped bat," because of its large, somewhat drooping lower lip. It is just possible that, while fishing, the bat purses its mouth and in this way directs its chirps downward against the water surface. Its loud, modulated calls might produce a detectable echo from a minnow's swim bladder, and return in time for the bat's legs to break through the surface and seize a victim. *Noctilio* skims so close to a minnow's world that the short working distance for the call may offset the stupendous losses in sound energy on two trips through the surface film.

Bats, like human beings, get tired. At such times or when not yet fully awakened for the night, they often blunder into obstacles avoided easily by individuals of the same kind after rest or when fully alert. Even the most skillful of them will collide with a wire a fiftieth of an inch in diameter if it is stretched horizontally about one and a half inches above the water surface in a stock watering trough. Apparently the bats come down to drink by skimming over the tank and dropping the lower jaw just enough to pick up a sip or two of water. While strong echoes of their cries are reflecting to them from the liquid surface, they fail to detect the less intense echoes from the wire and strike it, tumbling into the water. They may swim to the edge and clamber out, or take off like float planes from the water surface itself.

Another explanation for these collisions has been offered recently. A bat lives long enough to form habits, which include flight paths through places found on earlier trips to be free of obstacles. Along these routes they are easily surprised by changes, and blunder into newly erected barriers despite the echoes that must come back to their ears from the continuous staccato chirps produced on every flight. Apparently habit is too strong for a bat to believe its ears. Inattention of this kind may well explain the number of bats which annually strike the Empire State Building with enough force to kill themselves.

Naturalists who have been studying the echolocation methods of bats are well aware that success is seldom one-sided. Bats have a wonderful method for finding and following flying insects in the dark, and control their wings in pursuit tactics far more adeptly than any bird can do. But some insects have counter measures that decrease the chance of a bat's pursuing them. Many moths are so covered with fuzzy scales that they reflect little sound.

Other moths, and at least some beetles, possess a double range of hearing. They use one range for sounds from mates; the second is sensitive to the cries of approaching bats. When the high-range hearing receives a stimulus or two, the insect folds its wings and plummets to the earth, presumably escaping from the bat before becoming a detected target.

Submarines and military aircraft now carry comparable detection devices, allowing the crew to know immediately when they come into the field of radar search equipment. Prompt measures can often mislead the distant radar operators and let the vehicle proceed without interference. This technique could have been based upon knowledge of the echolocation systems of bats and the avoidance procedures of insects. Actually, the engineers responsible for improving defense devices have ignored the animals in which comparable problems were solved long ago.

Bats are not alone in their use of echoes in finding their way about through the dark. Some of the mice and shrews show that they can do so on the ground, or on the special elevated runways with which psychologists test an animal's ability to learn a maze. Seemingly these terrestrial creatures also utter ultrasonic cries, and detect their position according to the directions from which familiar echoes are received. In the wilds, the echoes would come from stones and tree trunks. Even the absence of an echo—the criterion by which a bat finds the opening to a cave or cranny—can be meaningful if vision is poor or the light too dim.

Anyone who has pet birds flying freely in the house knows how easily they can be caught as soon as the room is dark. Actually, until the 1950's, no one suspected that any bird could find its way without using its eyes. Certainly no owl has this ability. Yet two different types are now known to nest in completely dark parts of caves, guiding themselves to their roosts by echoes of their own clicking sounds.

The largest of these feathered cave dwellers is the oil bird *Steatornis*, found in suitable areas from Peru eastward through Venezuela into the Guianas in northern South America, and on the island of Trinidad. To meet such unusual birds, we clambered along an overgrown trail in the mountains of the island, carrying a portable metal ladder with which to enter and explore the cave. Rucksacks and pockets bulged with flashlights and flash equipment for our cameras, making a tumble on the slippery ground particularly hazardous.

Our diary, written up later that day, records the following:

> Oil birds evidently disturbed by our entry into high narrow cave; began flying about, but not going far toward light in entrance before turning back; squawking, screeching, clucking sounds almost deafened us. Birds surprisingly hawklike, each with wing spread of about three feet; chocolate brown with many large white spots; sturdy-looking beaks slightly downturned at tip; reddish eyeshine in light of flashlamps. Maneuver easily within confines of cave, or cling to almost vertical walls, pairs often side by side; nests high up, wherever a jutting point of rock provides a small horizontal surface. Clamor ceased whenever our lights turned off; then only swish of soft wings, breezes as birds passed close, and irregular repetitious clicking, high-pitched but quite audible.

These were the echo-producing calls, at a pitch close to seven thousand vibrations per second.

Oil birds roost by day and feed at night, hovering while they gather the fruit of various trees. They swallow the plumlike products of many different palms, including the commercial oil palm, but regurgitate the armored seeds. Seedlings from these soon sprout in the darkness of the home cave, only to die from lack of light. We found palm seeds even in the shallow mud nests high on the cave walls, and could distinguish enough from the size and markings to know that many of the local palms were represented. Yet the diet is so rich in oils that the birds themselves and their squabs are fat. Native people, for whom the price of a gallon of kerosene is a major expenditure, go into the oil-bird caves with torches and take both young and adults to render for the fat, which can be burned as a fuel. It is ironical that birds which assiduously avoid the light should yield the oil for dispelling darkness in the homes of man.

The other cave-dwelling birds, which have been discovered to be able to find their way by the echoes of their
own cries, are swallowlike swiftlets (*Callocalia*) of southern
India to Australia. The nests they construct entirely of
viscous saliva deep in the caves have become famous as the
chief ingredient of bird's-nest soup. The swiftlets themselves feed by day on flying insects, and sleep at night in the
same secluded places where bats spend the sunny hours. At
dawn and at sunset the birds and bats trade sleeping sites,
as though one worked on the day shift and the other the
night. The birds, however, use echolocating cries within
our audible spectrum. When in darkness they produce
calls described as resembling "those made by a child's
rapidly rotated ratchet toy," the clicks following one another at a rate of from five to ten per second.

Echoes are important also to water animals. Toothed
whales and porpoises, which are so well adapted to life in
the oceans that they outswim and eat fishes and squids,
communicate by audible grunts and ultrasonic whistles.
They are adept, too, at locating and identifying food by
echolocation, employing essentially the same methods as
man has invented recently and named "SOFAR" ("SOund
Fixing And Ranging"), sonar and echo sounding—the
principle of the fathometer.

Water conducts sound well. It absorbs far less energy
from the signal in a given distance than does a comparable
route through air. Yet it is scarcely an ideal medium for
echolocation methods, since sound vibrations are conducted through it almost five times as rapidly as through
air. A tone of middle C in water has a wave length of
235 inches, not 51 as in air. Yet the rule regarding reflection
holds for underwater sounds too: a surface must be several
times as broad as the wave length of a sound to reflect it
well. Underwater, a middle-C tone would scarcely echo
from anything smaller than the *Queen Elizabeth* or the
bottom. To use echoes, an aquatic animal is limited either
to detection of very large obstacles or to very high-
pitched sounds. Whales and porpoises rely upon cries in
the ultrasonic range, for which man has had detection
tools only in recent years.

These animals have another handicap—an inherited

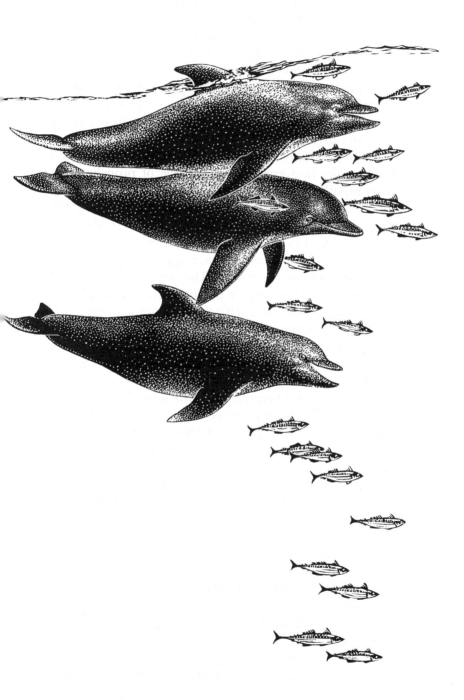

one. Whales and porpoises are mammals. Their ears are like ours in one respect: they contain small bones serving as levers of a translating mechanism, turning vibrations in an eardrum affected by sounds in air into vibrations of the fluid in the inner ear. As recently as fifty million years ago, their ancestors had legs and led an amphibious existence along the coasts, apparently escaping into the sea when pursued on land. Ears useful in air no longer suited a whale once it took to the water permanently and began extensive diving.

During the millennia while the animals' tails spread horizontally into great flukes capable of propelling the body rapidly, the evolutionary process affected their ears too. Probably as a protection from underwater noise, the ear openings shrank to the diameter of a lead pencil or less. The passageways also became filled with a waxy ear stopple—a plug in which annual rings can be found, indicating the age of the whale. The wax conducts sound vibrations from the water to the three leverlike little bones of the middle ear, just as effectively as our open passageways and eardrums do in air.

In the whale, at the same time, the air-filled space around the ear bones enlarged until it surrounded the sensitive inner ear itself, isolating it acoustically from the body. Much of the space became filled with a firm foam serving a dual role. The foam protects the whale's ear from pressure when the animal dives to a depth of as much as three thousand feet, where the surrounding water pushes against the ear stopple with a force of three-quarters of a ton to the square inch. Foam is also a wonderful sound-proofing material between the ear and the whale's great body, helping the whale to pay attention only to sound vibrations coming by way of its wax plugs.

All of these recent discoveries on the importance of echoes to living things show how much man might have learned from his animal neighbors if he had taken the time to interest himself in them. The fact that bats must be free to chirp and to hear if they are to dodge obstacles in the dark was proved experimentally and described in print by the Italian Lazzaro Spallanzani in 1793. The hypothesis that echoes serve bats in navigating without light was offered by the Englishman H. Hartridge in 1920. Between the 1920's and 1945, nearly three billion dollars were spent by the United States alone in solving problems of echo-location; other military powers invested vast sums. Yet in all those years just three people were devoting time—and only part time—to finding out how bats use echoes, as bats have been doing successfully for some fifty million years. Two of the three were graduate students, and the other man—a Dutch zoologist—was greatly hampered in research by the German occupation of his country.

Now that the naturalist, the biophysicist and the military man have come closer together in investigating the possibilities in ccholocation with ultrasonic waves, even applications to medicine are growing. A vibrating crystal, sending forth a high-pitched sound from its position on the surface of the human body, can provide the basis for informative echoes from normal and abnormal boundaries between organs deep inside. The new diagnostic tool offers some of the advantages of X-rays, without endangering children still to be conceived.

As is so characteristic of advances in science, new questions arise faster than old ones are answered. Do echoes guide a bat migrating between Canada and Central America, or a whale on the route Herman Melville described for the white whale Moby Dick? Do fish in the endless night of the ocean abysses maintain their depths within close limits by sounding signals echoed back to them from the bottom and the surface?

In fitting each of these new discoveries into its proper perspective, we are laying the basis too for future practical applications, whether in helping a blind man fit comfortably into a primarily visual world, or in aiding an engineer to reduce noise—allowing privacy in an era of growing human population.

II

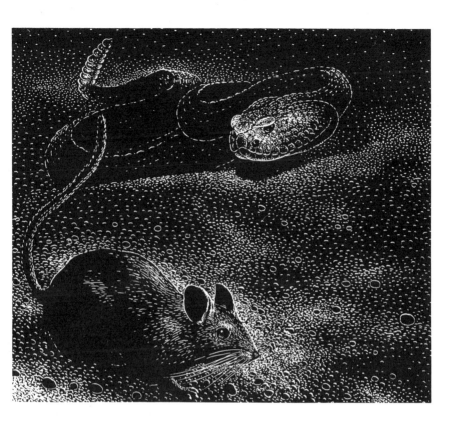

8. *Hot or Cold?*

AMONG THE hazards a skin diver faces, we think first of hungry sharks, slashing barracudas, stealthy octopuses or stinging corals. Rarely do we realize the far commoner danger from sudden exhaustion due to wastage of body heat into cold water. Yet skin divers must guard against this with special care, for their skins soon cease to remind them that they are continuing to lose energy. Watchmakers offer an underwater alarm to shake the diver's wrist at a predetermined time, for it is easy to forget that our whole judgment of temperature becomes severely biased by recent experience. Usually we are aware of this briefly as we wade into water, where only the skin wetted most recently warns us of the ocean's chill or of the heat we are gaining from a tub bath. We quickly grow accustomed to the temperature of our new surroundings.

Ordinarily we can rely upon our finger tips to caution us if a cup of coffee is too hot to drink. The skin of our grasping surfaces is a thicker insulation than lines the mouth. However, after touching something warm or cool, several minutes are required for the skin on the fingers to become neutral again. If we want to test the baby's bottle to see if the milk is too hot or too cool, we press the glass against the hairless side of the forearm, preferably near the elbow. There the skin is fairly sensitive, and less likely to have been in biasing contact with nearby objects. Similarly, we touch the back of our fingers or the heel of the hand against a child's brow when we are anxious to judge if a fever has developed.

In many primitive societies, a mother or the medicine man looks for a different proof of health. So long as lice are present on the head, the child or oldster is in good condition. If a person develops a fever, these parasites grow uncomfortable and shift to a new victim. Similarly, if the body temperature falls a few degrees, the vermin desert it. Whether on man or other warm-blooded animals, lice and fleas appear to possess good internal thermometers. The spread of bubonic plague, in fact, is credited to the rapid transfer of fleas from fevered rats to other rats or to man, creating epidemics of the dread disease.

One of the personal differences among people, making some of us almost immune to infections carried by external parasites, lies in the amount of heat we radiate. Usually the same person attracts chiggers, fleas, mosquitoes and other pests, and could be regarded as "parasite prone." When out walking in the evening with a companion, he who glows with inner warmth becomes the center of a cloud of mosquitoes—a distinction that is rarely appreciated. The insects settle and begin to bite. The victim slaps at them, raising the already high skin temperature by this exertion. More and more mosquitoes buzz to the scene.

All this time, no insects bother the victim's chilly companion, who is surprised at all the commotion. Until shown the bodies of mashed mosquitoes, the unbitten person may disbelieve that they are around. Even when walking alone, such people usually attract few parasites. Yet, if they have a fever or if they run awhile and get their skin temperatures well above their usual range, they too become parasite prone.

Apparently Charles Darwin was one of these warm-skinned people. He reported in his diary of the *Beagle* voyage being attacked by large bloodsucking bugs (*Triatoma*) in South America on the night of March 26, 1835. Not until 1959, however, did anyone point out the probable connection between this event and the prolonged invalidism Darwin suffered following his return to England. The symptoms of his later illness correspond well with those of a chronic case of Chagas' disease, a trypanosome infection now known to be transmitted through the bite of this bug.

It is tempting to wonder whether, had Darwin not been parasite prone, he might have returned home uninfected to a vigorous life in the London suburbs, with no time to mull over his personal observations and those in the scientific literature. What gave Darwin the opportunity to marshal the wealth of factual information in *The Origin of Species*, giving the idea of natural selection to the world? We can't shrug and point out that, if Darwin had not done the work, Alfred Russel Wallace was ready with the same concept. Wallace too lacked the time to think out the causative force in evolution until he was laid up in Ternate with a prolonged bout of malaria, brought to him by a mosquito. He was parasite prone too!

Despite any refutation from history, most of us are firmly convinced that days spent being sick are entirely wasted. If we cannot cease being warm-blooded and parasite prone, is there any way to protect ourselves from the annoyance of the bites and against lost time? One method was discovered by keeping a tally on the biting flies settling on dummy men warmed by internal heaters. Dummies are far more attractive to the insects when garbed in black or dark materials which radiate heat well. The dull finish of crepes and cottons was particularly effective. White or light-colored clothing, especially if shiny (like satin or nylon), actually reduced the likelihood of attack by diminishing the radiation of heat energy.

Supposedly a white skin, or white clothing such as Caucasoid people often wear in the tropics, serves as protection from mosquitoes and many other insects that find their victims through the heat they radiate. But white skin or white garments form conspicuous targets for other insects, such as horse flies and deer flies, which hunt by sight, and for stinging insects, such as wasps. The Indians of Darien province in Panama are more concerned about being seen than being detected by mosquitoes. They paint their light skins black, explaining that fewer insects attack them when their bodies blend with the jungle shadows. It is possible that so long as these people stay in the shade they also remain cooler by radiating more heat through their blackened skin.

In finding warm skin, a female mosquito relies upon her heat-sensitive antennae. Although these feelers themselves are less than an eighth of an inch long on a malaria-carrying *Anopheles* and still shorter on the yellow-fever mosquito *Aédes*, the insect can turn until both antennae are receiving the same amount of radiant heat. Then, by flying straight ahead for many yards, if necessary, the mosquito arrives at the warm-blooded victims. Male mosquitoes, by contrast, sip only plant juices and die soon after mating.

At night, enough radiant heat passes through glass windows or screens from a warm house to attract female mosquitoes flying by outdoors. Sometimes so many of them hover before the small openings in a window screen that the whining sound of their wings is audible inside. Generally these insects are so persistent that they discover any narrow crack and enter. Once in the bedroom where people are sleeping, the mosquitoes detect radiant warmth emanating from human bodies and press the attack farther.

If a female mosquito injures both of her antennae and loses the use of her heat-sensitive hunting system, she can find a blood meal only by accident. The same is true of the inch-long "giant bedbugs" of South and Central America, which carry Chagas' disease. These huge bugs can manage, however, with one antenna. They will point the one toward a glass rod just a few degrees warmer than the surroundings and pursue it, detecting a contrast in temperature between the far and the near end of the antenna.

So delicate a sensitivity to heat challenges man's engineering ingenuity. For space capsules and other devices he is constantly seeking to reduce the size and weight of his instruments, to "miniaturize" them. But the only feature capable of revealing the direction from which heat radiations come is the decrease in intensity corresponding to greater distance from the heat source. Where is there any significant distance from one end of a mosquito to the other, let alone between the ends of its antennae? No pair of man's miniature thermometers will indicate a difference in heat received if they are so close together.

As a radiant-heat-sensing system, an antenna is not the most remarkable pattern man might imitate. With no antennae whatever, a chicken mite less than 1/32 of an inch long shows at least as accurate sensitivity to the direction from which it receives radiant heat. At nightfall these diminutive creatures creep from crannies in the hen house and seek warm blood when the domestic fowl settle on their perches. Toward dawn, when the rooster crows and the hens grow restive, the mites leave again and find their crevices for the day. Perhaps in this way they avoid being flung off during a hen's daytime dust bath. Possibly the mites' departure is merely a sign of their intolerance of the fowl's daytime skin temperature, which rises as ours does when we awaken for the day.

The migration of chicken mites to warm objects at night can produce some odd results. In one hen house, so many of these parasites invaded an electric clock hanging on the wall that they interfered with the running of the mechanism. Even the stalled clock emitted heat. Around dawn, however, the mites left and the clock started again. Perhaps an early ray of sun struck the clock and raised its temperature a few degrees, driving out the mites. The hen-house owner took the clock to a repair shop, only to be told that nothing was wrong. Still the clock lost many hours every night. Since clock repairmen work by day, a great deal of sleuthing was needed to learn the true cause of the difficulty.

The radiant heat to which mites and mosquitoes respond is actually an invisible kind of light—the infrared beyond the red in the complete solar spectrum. It emanates strongly from a hot flatiron and feebly from a warm-bodied animal or a running clock motor. At night, infrared can be shone on objects from a special lamp covered by a filter that holds back any light to which our eyes would respond. A scene so irradiated is visible only through an infrared telescope, such as the "snooperscope" and "sniperscope" developed originally for military use. The smallest of these devices yet announced, together with its electric-power supply, is about the size of a large pair of field glasses and weighs at least as much. Larger versions have been incorporated into anti-aircraft rockets such as the "Sidewinder," which seeks out its target by homing on the more intense infrared from hot engines and exhaust fumes. Infrared telescopes serve also in "weather-eye" satellites hundreds of miles above the ground, where they can produce pictures from the infrared in sunshine, reflected through the earth's hazy atmosphere. Through the wizardry of infrared image tubes, television circuits, video tape and short-wave radio, these pictures can be transmitted back to earth, extending man's senses in new dimensions.

After these devices sensitive to radiant heat had been invented, biologists discovered that for millions of years rattlesnakes and other pit vipers have been quietly using a strictly comparable method while hunting for prey after dark. Between the nostril and the eye on each side of a pit viper's head are two conical craters lined with special cells sensitive to radiant heat (infrared). Since heat energy of this type travels like light in straight lines, the pit organs receive radiations from only certain directions. If they were eyes we could speak of their field of view, and comment that the snake had binocular vision. Since they are pit organs, the best we can do is describe their fields of sensitivity as overlapping straight ahead of the snake and at a specific distance. This proves to be the striking distance when the snake is coiled to best advantage.

While hunting, the pit viper crawls along slowly, scanning the ground and low bushes for anything cooler or warmer than the general surroundings. A mere thousandth of a degree Fahrenheit is enough difference in temperature to alert the snake. Little by little it silently approaches the object — a frog chilled by evaporation of moisture from its skin, a slumbering bird or perhaps a man in a sleeping bag. Using its overlapping conical fields of heat sensitivity, the snake can learn when it has come within striking distance, and also a great deal about the size and position of potential prey.

It seems unlikely that pit vipers strike offensively at animals too large to be useful as food. Their pit organs permit them, of course, to strike defensively at a passing human foot or any other part of a warm-blooded animal thrust in their direction. One of the rare fatalities in the United States occurred a few years ago in New England when a girl was too embarrassed to say anything after being bitten in the dark. She had gone beyond the glow of the campfire to "attend to a call of nature," and was struck on a large warm area where a tourniquet could scarcely be applied. However, packing the wound in ice until she could be taken to a competent physician would almost certainly have saved her life. So good is the chance of rescue through medical treatment — if given in time — that the number of people in Anglo-America dying from snake bite each year is smaller than the total killed by lightning while playing golf! Yet we are so day-minded that we dread any snake that can locate us in complete darkness.

Our own sense organs are nowhere nearly so responsive to heat and cold as those in the pit viper's head. We have a double set. About 150,000 of them alert us to loss of heat to "cold" objects, and about 16,000 to entry of heat from "hot" objects. The nerve endings sensitive to heat outflow lie mostly within a fiftieth of an inch of the skin surface; about two-thirds of them are associated with the openings of the sweat glands. The sense organs responding to the inflow of heat reside deeper in the skin, where they are somewhat insulated from external changes in temperature; they react more slowly than the cold endings. If we damage the insulation and admit heat through a cut in the skin, things that would be bearably hot cause a painful stinging sensation at once.

Heat receptors are most numerous in the skin of the finger tips, nose and bend of the elbow. Cold receptors abound particularly in the skin of the upper lip, nose,

chin, chest, forehead and fingers. Curiously, both types
are lacking in the eye; it is the one area of the body insensitive to heat and cold.

Our finest warmth-sensing system is a thermostat in the
hypothalamus of the brain, close to the pituitary gland and
to branches of the main artery bringing blood from the
heart to the head. No matter where the body gains or loses
heat, the change is felt promptly. Even drinking a cup of
hot tea or a glass of cold water alters the temperature of the
blood reaching the heat-sensing center. Taking these
liquids may have no effect on a clinical thermometer
tucked under the tongue. Only a delicate thermometer applied carefully to the eardrum will record these changes,
and then not before the brain has acted upon them in
regulating both the body's heat production and its dissipation.

Our experience with body temperature is usually limited
to the information we get from a clinical thermometer: a
normal range between 96 and 99 degrees. The skin surface,
however, averages close to 81 degrees F. A naked savage
remains in thermal equilibrium with his environment if the
air temperature is in the low 80's. Usually we add clothes
or choose lighter ones to maintain the temperature of protected skin surfaces somewhat above 81 degrees, and depend upon greater loss of heat (and lower surface temperatures) over our exposed hands and face.

We take our stabilized body temperature so much for
granted that we are likely to overlook the energy we spend
to keep ourselves from becoming inactive in cold weather
and endangered by hot. Only mammals and birds increase
glandular activity and muscular tension — to the stage
of shivering, if necessary — to produce more heat when
the blood temperature is threatening to fall. Only "warm-
blooded" creatures sweat and pant vigorously, cooling
themselves through evaporation of water, when dissipation of body heat is slower than its production and the
blood temperature threatens to rise.

Through inability to maintain body warmth at a constant level despite variations in the temperature of the
environment, "cold-blooded" animals must be opportunists. They can enjoy full activity only when the weather

is warm enough for the chemical reactions of life to proceed at a brisk pace. Hot weather from which they cannot escape is fatal to them.

Cold-blooded animals in water often behave as though they were able to judge the temperature. The little water flea *Daphnia*, which swims as though dancing by jerks of its long antennae in the surface waters of fresh ponds over much of the world, survives for about three and a half months at a chilly 46 degrees F. At a sultry 81 it dies after nearly as many weeks. The total number of its heartbeats is almost identical at the two temperatures. In the cold water, however, *Daphnia* cannot reproduce. At 81 degrees, a newly mature individual begins releasing close to fifty young every four days until about six broods have gone out on their own. At this temperature, *Daphnia* also tends to seek deeper, cooler water. The animal has no need to measure the warmth of its pond. Its whole rate of living is affected because most chemical reactions are speeded up by a rise in temperature.

Is an animal cold-blooded because its nervous system allows it to make no distinction between cold and warm, or because the creature has no way to alter the temperature of its body into a more comfortable range? Does a fish feel hot or cold? Recently some goldfish at Harvard University gave the answer when they were provided with a lever which, when pressed, caused cold water to squirt for a second into their bowl, lowering their environmental temperature about half a degree Fahrenheit. After a little training had acquainted a goldfish with the importance of the lever, the fish would thrust its head through a hole in a Plexiglas shield to reach the bar and press hard as soon as the environment had been warmed to 91 degrees. Some individual goldfishes excelled in lever-pressing, and kept the temperature of their watery world between 95 and 97 — well below the 106 degrees that soon is fatal to them. Trained fish introduced into water at 106 degrees worked frantically, saving themselves from heat death. They pressed the lever repeatedly until the environmental temperature changed into the 95- to 97-degree range, as though this were comfortable. Apparently all a cold-blooded fish needs is a way to adjust its living conditions; it has its own internal thermometer.

Animals on land seem able to find suitable warmth more easily than those in water. In the daytime ants carry their eggs and young into spaces below boards and flat rocks heated by the sun, where they will develop faster than in the cool chambers deep in the soil. Bears find the ants by pulling the covers aside. Nocturnal hunters, such as skunks and raccoons, have less chance to do so, for as soon as the sun sinks toward the horizon the ants take their charges below again and do not return until the middle of the following morning.

In providing their young with temperature-conditioned brood chambers, some insects have gone far beyond opportunism. In arid and semi-arid highlands of Australia, Asia, Africa, South and Central America, soft-bodied termites build almost cement-hard nests above ground, where the heat of the sun can speed the growth processes of the insects within. At the same time, these thin-skinned, pale-bodied creatures remain protected from dry air. Some of the mounds are twelve feet in diameter and twenty feet high. Those in northern Australia are famous because they have the form of thin vanes oriented accurately to face east and west. Presumably the mounds absorb less heat from the noonday sun, but extend the day for the brood within by picking up radiant heat soon after dawn and until near sunset.

Man's own adventures in producing artificial climates have gone several steps beyond the achievements of ants and termites. However, our friends the honeybees manage in their simple way to cool the hive as well as heat it, according to a temperature sense hidden somewhere within them. On hot days, almost all of the workers leave the hive and rest outdoors in the shade, where heat from their bodies will not raise the temperature of the growing young and of the food stores. A few bees stand in the doorway to the hive, fanning their wings continuously and driving air into the darkness within. Additional workers bring water, and regurgitate it at the tops of the combs. It evaporates while dripping down the vertical surfaces, and helps to cool the hive. In winter, by contrast, the bees cluster on the comb. With vigorous body movements they generate heat. To continue this muscular work they must make frequent visits to the honey stores to obtain new cropfuls of energy-supplying food.

When you come to think about it, you cannot be certain that the familiar explanation for the bees' honey store is the correct one. How important are the reserves of concentrated nectar during the months when new generations of bees are being raised? The season of brood care corresponds to the time when nectar is plentiful in the fields. A modest store of honey would suffice to tide them over inclement weather, when the brood must be fed despite fog or rain that grounds all the workers on their beeports. The bulk of the honey store — or of some cheaper substitute the beekeeper furnishes after harvesting the loaded combs — is needed as the fuel source for winter labors, keeping the hive above 65 degrees F. even if the outside temperature falls to forty below zero. Would man have adopted the honeybee and Virgil have lauded its labors if it had not pioneered in keeping its quarters warm in winter — responding to its temperature sense?

A beehive serves both as a home for the colony and as a nursery for the queen's offspring. By having a dual role, a hive differs significantly from a bird's nest, which is simply an incubator used later as a cradle. Parent birds do not go "home" to the nest to spend a rainy day, or even to sleep unless there are young to be cared for. Only a few birds, in fact, have developed production-line methods for producing offspring, vaguely comparable to the system used in a beehive. These few, however, have become highly efficient, partly because the hatchlings require no care whatever after they escape from the egg, and partly because the beak of the male bird has become an incredibly good thermometer.

The birds that show these astonishing habits are the megapodes of Australia and New Guinea. Some of these big-footed turkey-sized megapodes are known as brush turkeys, mallee fowl and jungle fowl. The hen bird in many instances manages to lay a half-pound egg every four days for almost five months each year, which is quite a feat for a fowl weighing only about three and a half pounds. She is far too busy eating and producing eggs to spend time incubating them. Nor could her mate manage with nearly forty eggs per season except for the fact that he has become a specialist in operating an incubator.

At the beginning of the mating season, both members of a pair of megapodes co-operate in building a mound of earth as much as fifty feet in diameter and from fifteen to twenty feet high. Or the male may do the work alone, often rehabilitating an old mound from the year before. In each completed mound, he opens a large pit at the top and stocks it with wet vegetation. When this is covered with sand, fermentation liberates heat, warming the sand. Somehow the bird manages to collect just the correct amount of vegetation to produce a temperature close to 92 degrees F. a few inches below the surface. In this warm sand, the female lays her eggs under the male's constant supervision.

Several times a day, the cock megapode thrusts his beak into the sand near the eggs and appears to measure the temperature. If it is too cool, he brings more sand and adds another layer of insulation. If it is too warm, he opens holes to the rotting vegetable matter. In the very early morning, he may pull the surface sand down to the sides of the mound, where it will take on the chill of the adjacent ground, and then drag it up over the nest area, where it will cool the layer covering the eggs.

We think of the actions of birds as arising almost exclusively from instincts — ready-made responses inherited by each new generation. How can instinctive behavior be so adjustable in a cock megapode? Can this be the ultimate in a gradual adaptation, beginning with tropical birds that merely covered their eggs with damp leaves as a means of giving the clutch some camouflage while the parents were away feeding? Whatever the evolutionary history, local conditions are used by the megapodes to an astonishing degree. In some areas, where the soil is warm from thermal springs or recent volcanic activity, the megapodes have adopted this natural incubator and undertaken to control the heat loss from the ground to keep their buried eggs developing at approximately 92 degrees.

This temperature must have some magic about it, for the megapodes achieve 92 degrees in both the coolest part of their range and the most tropical. It is within a degree, moreover, of the temperature found in nests of wild American birds of many kinds. Scientists have established these facts by thrusting delicate metallic thermometers (thermocouples) into eggs while they were being incubated. When a robin left the nest, the clutch in some instances dropped to a chilly 44 degrees on a windy spring day. Then the parent returned, fluffed out her feathers over the shells, and the development of the young inside progressed a little farther.

More than the presence of the parent affects egg temperatures. Direct sun or a strong wind penetrates the insulation of the nest and raises or lowers the heat levels inside the eggs by many degrees. Even the location of an egg in the clutch is important. One mallard duck was most solicitous in her care of eighteen eggs. Whenever the egg containing the tattletale thermocouple was in the center of the cluster, its temperature rose into the nineties. At the outer edge of the group the heat level wavered between the sixties and seventies. All this shows how important it is for the parent bird to keep rearranging the incubating eggs, so that each will hatch within a few days of the others.

We can see a striking correspondence between the responses of animals to changes in temperature and those among human beings. The majority of people are like the cock megapode bird in doing their best to adjust to whatever local conditions and weather happen to be. Instead of opening holes to the fermenting vegetation or pulling cool sand up on the nest mound, they meet hot days by encouraging shade trees, putting up awnings, closing the windows after each cool night, or installing air-conditioning. When the weather turns chilly, we don't haul additional earth over the house as insulation. But we may install storm windows and reach for the switch that starts the furnace.

People with no firm ties to a given place may be more like the Canada geese. With the arrival of unwelcome chill, they drift southward to Florida or California. Some of them hurry north again in spring, although few are as insistent as the geese, which follow the thaws all the way to the Arctic, remaining on the northbound edge of the 35-degree isotherm for as much as two thousand miles.

Those of us who make our living in the intemperate Temperate Zone often forget that a few places in the world offer idyllic temperatures all year. Many animals seem to have taken advantage of this fact. In 1939, Professor Otto Rahn published a tally he had made: 2,076 species of mammals and 2,785 kinds of reptiles living in the tropics, as against 948 species of mammals and 335 of reptiles living in the changeable temperate zones to the north and south. Most of these differences represent faster evolution in the tropics than in cooler climates, partly because of larger numbers of generations annually. Only a few of these kinds of mammals and reptiles stay where they do because of preferences shown after spreading over a whole range of temperatures and multiplying fastest in some favored region.

Sailors have far more opportunity to choose on the basis of wide experience. It was no accident that led the mutineers aboard H.M.S. *Bounty* to settle on Pitcairn Island after exchanging their commander, Admiral William Bligh, for a boatload of ladies from tropical isles. Pitcairn is about as far south of the equator as Miami is north of it. Similarly, Herman Melville and Robert Louis Stevenson and E. H. Paul Gauguin felt free to choose. They picked out tropical paradises and proceeded to make them famous.

So far, no one has succeeded in emulating animals in another way they respond to large changes in temperature. And yet the question grows ever more important: can man be induced to hibernate, in the same sense that groundhogs and various bats do every year? Real advantages could be found. The world's food supply might support twelve billion people fairly well if, each year, every individual took a four-month turn at being awake and active, producing the food and enjoying it. For the other eight months, each person could be dormant, chilled and only very slowly using up food reserves set aside for this form of survival.

Engineers charged with the design of interplanetary space ships are even more enthusiastic about rocketing astronauts at least part of the way in a chilled and dormant state. Logistic problems would be simplified enormously through reduced requirements for oxygen, food, water, absorption of carbon dioxide, disposal of wastes, maintenance of cabin temperature in a narrow range, and entertainment too. Moreover, the temporary immunity to harmful radiations shown by hibernating animals might have a counterpart in man. The astronauts in their chilling chamber might pass through belts of dangerous rays, with life-saving treatment for radiation damage deferred until a later, more convenient time, after arrival somewhere.

Already great strides have been made in this direction. People who are unable to tolerate conventional anesthetics can be prepared for surgery by being chilled uniformly, carefully and rapidly. All sensations disappear, and the rate of blood flow is lowered. Yet, when rewarmed with equal care, the patients develop no complications and recall none of the experience.

When a person is cooled uniformly below 94 degrees F., vision and hearing disappear. Below 85 degrees the normal thermostat mechanism ceases to call for activity that would raise body temperature, and the patient is utterly dependent upon the attending physicians. The pupils open widely; sensation has vanished; the pulse continues at about forty per minute, as compared with the normal seventy to seventy-five; blood pressure is low and steady. Respiratory movements too cease at about 80 degrees. Surgery is done ordinarily just below this temperature — at 77. An artificial respirator is adjusted to fill the lungs with pure oxygen and empty them again perhaps thirty times a minute. When the surgeons finish their work, the body temperature is returned to normal by even heating. At 80 degrees, respiratory impulses appear. The pulse returns at 86, and blood pressure again becomes measurable. At 90 degrees the body thermostat takes hold. At 94, vision and hearing return.

Dogs have been chilled much more than this. At about 50 degrees, the heart stops. But if artificial means are used for circulating the blood, little need for oxygen can be found. At 39 degrees, no difference can be detected in the oxygen content of blood entering and leaving organs. Hibernating animals, by contrast, continue to need oxygen all the way to the freezing point. They maintain a slow heart action and breathe at intervals. At any temperature above freezing, moreover, they can awaken themselves. With as much as a fiftyfold increase in heat production, they raise their body temperature perhaps 53 degrees in three hours. Curiously, a hibernator's fat is different too. It remains liquid to very low temperatures, whereas human fat solidifies at about 45 degrees.

Unless the astronauts could be made to hibernate in some kind of an automatic cabinet that would return them to normal temperature safely, the cost of care would far outweigh any gains that might be found in rocketing them in a chilled state. Even then, disadvantages may turn up, features still beyond our imagination. One of them might be a human equivalent of the color pattern in Himalayan strains of domestic rabbits. So long as this particular breed is maintained in quarters at 81 degrees or higher, the rabbits are pure white. At significantly lower temperatures, the tips of ears, of the paws, of the nose and of a saddle-shaped area on the back all produce black pigment in a characteristic pattern.

The difference between the all-white Himalayan rabbit and the one with black markings is due entirely to the temperature of the skin at the time when pigment and hair are being produced. The normal blood circulation is not rapid enough to keep these areas warmed into the range at which formation of black pigment is inhibited. Comparable results can be obtained by keeping an ice pack against any area of the rabbit's skin prior to periods when new fur appears.

The hairs on a man's scalp and face grow every day. Who knows what pattern they might develop on an astronaut kept for a few weeks at hibernating temperatures? Already biologists have wondered why man comes in assorted colors, but never covered with hair in contrasting patches like those we see on guinea pigs and cattle. Perhaps a cold treatment will provide the missing types. They might become useful as a sort of personal camouflage in the bizarre environment of some distant planet.

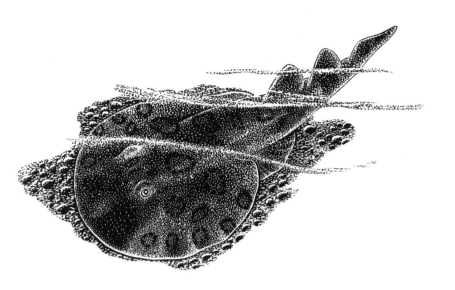

9. *Shocking Information*

EVER SINCE man became sentient, he has been aware that when anything struck him forcefully on the eye he experienced a sensation of light as well as of pain. Even the shock of a blow on the head may provide enough mechanical stimulation for the eyes to report that they see "stars." Yet, until the late 1820's, no scientific explanation was available. Then the outstanding German physiologist Johannes Müller, still in his twenties, suddenly realized that the destination of a nerve determines the meaning of its message. The part of the brain to which the optic nerve goes from the eye can interpret messages only as sight, although particularly compelling messages may spill over into other areas of the brain and be felt as pain.

Nerve messages from the eye, the nose and other parts of the body are all of one type. They consist of electro-chemical changes sweeping along as swiftly as four hundred feet a second, always as discrete pulses lasting about a ten-thousandth of a second. If a stimulus is intense, the impulses may follow one another every thousandth of a second. Or the nerve may transmit them at greater intervals, often in bursts of activity that give the brain added information in a simple code.

Although a nerve impulse is not a current of electricity (and hence does not travel at the speed of light—186,000 miles per second), all nerve cells can be induced to conduct impulses if stimulated electrically. Since 1943 it has been clear that identical sparks of high-voltage electricity striking the human skin singly at different points can arouse in the brain the sensations of warmth, cold, pain, pressure and "touch" depending upon which nerve endings the spark affects. The same stimuli on the tongue give the additional mental impressions of bitter, salty, sour or sweet, according to the individual receptor systems excited.

We cannot actually feel electricity. None of our sense organs is adapted to alert our brain that we are being stimulated in this way. Instead, each sense organ is especially sensitive to some other type of stimulus. In relation to these special sensitivities, our brain interprets the messages along the nerves associated with each particular sense organ. The messages themselves are all of a single type, and similar to those that travel from the brain to the muscles when we deliberately wish to move. They have nothing to do with the tingling sensation or the sudden cramping pain we feel from an electric shock, which excites our muscles into violent contraction. Normal nerve messages induce activity with far less expenditure of energy and much better control.

Our ability to tolerate an electric shock has been put to use recently by a clockmaker in Nuremberg, Germany. He offered for sale a shocking alarm clock for deaf people. The strength of the electric shock delivered at the desired hour could be regulated according to the amount needed to awaken the sleeper.

Perhaps some similar shocking attachment would be a money-saving improvement for the new radar-detection devices that motorists are offered as accessories. Intended to buzz a warning to a speeding driver as soon as he comes within range of a radar trap set by highway police, the device often fails to get attention in time. Not only is the human body insensitive to radar signals themselves, but it may also ignore audible signals a while if they are competing with conversation or a program on the car radio. Any delay in pushing down on the brake pedal lets the radar operator complete his measurement and radio to a second officer in a pickup cruise car to issue a summons for the traffic violation. With a more insistent message, such as an electric shock might convey, the erring motorist would be more likely to slow his car to a legal speed before it came fully into range of the radar meter.

Our lack of special sense organs for electricity is matched by a general unawareness that every active gland cell and any contracting muscle produces electricity. The amount is too slight to affect nerves in the vicinity. Yet if the nerve to a surviving leg muscle is laid across an exposed beating heart, the leg will twitch in time with the heartbeat. A human heart generates enough electrical currents in the body to produce rhythmic changes of from $1/500$ to $1/100$ of a volt at the surface of the chest. These changes can be amplified and recorded as an electrocardiogram, from which a cardiologist can tell whether the heart is beating normally. Minute currents due to brain activity are popularly known as brain waves; they can be detected similarly on the scalp, and recorded in amplified form as an electroencephalogram. They are valuable clues in detecting damage to the brain, and have recently been put to a new use in learning whether messages intended to instruct deaf children are actually getting into each child's head and being recognized.

The small amounts of electricity generated by active cells usually have no known effect. Yet if electrical changes are introduced into the environment of many nonhuman types of life, from single-celled animals to fishes, they cause definite responses. For about fifty years, it has been known that the minute slipper animalcule *Paramecium* could detect the direction of an electric current, showing a sensitivity we do not possess. Here in the organization of a microscopic cell is a sense with no imaginable use. Countless paramecia have been watched in drops of pond water from the opposite sides of which wires led to a storage battery. These creatures always swim toward the negative connection. Even though this astonishing sense seems meaningless to the single cell, man has seen in it a principle he might apply to the breeding of animals.

The male reproductive cells of mammals react to direct electric currents, but male-producing sperms are drawn one way and female-producing sperms in the opposite direction. This difference has been used both experimentally and commercially in artificial insemination, where animal breeders prefer young of one sex to be born in their flocks or herds. It is far from a perfect method, but significantly better than chance.

A much more reliable use for electricity has been found in separating fishes, whose sensitivity varies greatly from one kind to another. Trout and salmon, like many other game fishes and economically valuable ones, skillfully avoid pulsating electromagnetic fields from picketlike wires hung as a barrier in a river. A V-shaped fence of this kind will deflect these jaw-bearing fishes while they are migrating upstream, and guide them into an inspection pen at the point of the V. There any harmful species can be removed before the others are allowed to proceed. By contrast, the jawless lampreys in upstream migration seem much less sensitive. They often bump into such barriers and get electrocuted.

During 1956, the United States and Canada invested nearly three million dollars in electric fences across streams flowing into Lakes Huron, Michigan and Superior, in an attempt to block the spawning migrations of parasitic lampreys and hence eliminate this destroyer of the fisheries in the Upper Great Lakes. Benefits from these measures may be expected after 1963. In the intervening years, young lampreys hatched from eggs deposited upstream in pre-barrier seasons will be descending unharmed past the barriers each spring and fall, to attack whatever large fishes they can find in the upper Great Lakes.

A series of discoveries made between 1956 and 1958 give reason for astonishment over the behavior of adult lampreys migrating in fresh water. Why should these creatures be so insensitive to electric barriers that they will bump into them, when almost identical lampreys in the sea find their victims through an electrical sensitivity suggesting underwater radar? Sea lampreys do become excited by the mere presence in the water of chemical compounds in minute quantities given off by their prey. This chemical sensitivity is not precise enough, however, to let them catch fishes except by accident. Their eyes are too degenerate to be useful. Instead, each excited sea lamprey emits brief electric pulses ("spike potentials"). Each momentary pulse consists of an electric current emerging from one area of the lamprey's body into the surrounding water, and back into other areas of the lamprey's skin. Apparently any change in the pattern with which the electric current returns is sensed by the lamprey. Ordinarily a change means that some object differing in electrical conductivity from plain water is within four inches of the lamprey's head. Often the object proves to be a fish upon which the lamprey can fasten its jawless sucker mouth and rasp a hole through to the victim's nourishing blood.

If electrical sensitivity is linked closely to hunting for prey, it is easier to explain why lampreys bump into electric barriers. Both the sea lampreys and those in the Great Lakes cease feeding when they become mature. They migrate into the upper reaches of streams, where they mate, discharge their milt or eggs, and die. After beginning their final fast, lampreys may simply cease to heed their sense organs having to do with electric currents. Another possibility is that, at any age, lampreys investigate every distortion of their pulsed electric currents — even barrier wires erected to electrocute them.

These discoveries of the lampreys' "sixth sense" came because scientists were anxious to learn all they could about lampreys, especially to determine why lampreys are so destructive to large fishes in fresh water but not to those in the sea. These parasites are no great problem to marine fisheries, except as ravagers of fishes held in nets and hence unable to escape.

Probably a healthy marine fish, possessing no greater electrical sensitivity than a freshwater one, detects an approaching sea lamprey while it still has time to escape. Lampreys may succeed in the ocean only in capturing sick, inattentive fishes. On this basis they would occupy a natural role in the marine environment comparable to that of wolves or lions on land. These carnivores eliminate chiefly the diseased and the aged; they rarely deplete the source of their food supply.

In fresh water, the contest between lampreys and jaw-bearing fishes is local and new on an evolutionary time scale. Lampreys, which belong to the most ancient group of animals with a backbone, seem to have remained exclusively marine until near the end of the great Ice Age. Then, with adjustments of the North American continent as it recovered from its burden of overlying ice, lampreys became landlocked in some freshwater lakes. These extended from Lake Champlain along the Vermont boundary to the Finger Lakes of upper New York State, and to Lake Ontario. It was the lampreys from Lake Ontario that spread, between 1935 and 1948, through man-made canals into the upper Great Lakes and ruined the fisheries industry there.

Jaw-bearing fishes originated in fresh waters where, until recently, they never had to contend with lampreys. Yet they show a sensitivity to electromagnetic fields that is adequate to let them dodge electric barriers. This adaptation, which seems valueless under natural conditions in fresh waters, may well have been highly important long ago when jaw-bearing fishes invaded the seas where lampreys were already well established.

For the electrical sensitivity of jaw-bearing fishes to warn them of the approach of lampreys in salt water, but not in fresh, is no paradox. Fresh water is notoriously poor as a conductor of electricity, whereas sea water is fairly good. Lampreys, however, might still use their electrical pulses profitably in fresh water while finding fishes as prey, even though detection would be at closer range than in the sea. In fresh water a lamprey actually would have an advantage in relying upon electromagnetic fields rather than on vision, for fresh waters are far more turbid than the oceans. Light penetrates to the bottom of only shallow lakes and rivers. Often fresh waters are so murky that eyes are almost useless a few feet below the surface; any fish depending on them is handicapped. Perhaps the poorer conduction of an electrical warning, coupled with the greater turbidity of fresh water, explains why fishes succumb to lampreys in lakes whereas those in the oceans escape.

The source of the lamprey's electricity remains to be discovered. So do the sense organs with which it detects changes in the pattern of pulsed electric currents through the surrounding water. However, electric organs in fishes have been known for almost two centuries. Charles Darwin puzzled over them, and remarked in his *Origin of Species* that "the electric organs of fishes offer another case of special difficulty; it is impossible to conceive by what steps these wondrous organs have been produced . . . they occur in only about a dozen fishes, of which several are widely remote in their affinities." He felt sure that the earliest ancestral fishes did not generate electricity. Yet how else could electric organs appear in such distantly related fishes?

Until 1958, offense and defense seemed the only uses of electric organs. Then, in an eel-like freshwater fish from Africa — one known to have feeble electric organs — a sensitivity to electromagnetic fields was discovered, comparable to that of the sea lamprey. In another African fish, a small sense organ was found close to the dorsal fin, responding to electrical pulses as brief as a ten-thousandth of a second. The knifefish *Eigenmannia* of warm waters along America's Atlantic coast proved to have an electric organ near the tip of the long tail. With this organ emitting pulses of electric current, the creature backs into small holes or uses the tail as a sort of probe with which to investigate objects in its surroundings. All of these new discoveries may modify our thinking about the sensory abilities of aquatic animals. Already they have filled in some of the gaps in knowledge which so perplexed Charles Darwin.

The nature of electric organs in fishes was recognized almost as soon as scientists identified electricity itself. For two thousand years previously, no one had been able to explain the ability of the square-fronted ray *Torpedo* to stun small fishes as prey. Aristotle described how this familiar denizen of the Mediterranean Sea "narcotizes the creatures that it wants to catch, overpowering them by the power of shock that is resident in its body, . . . This phenomenon has been actually observed in operation." *Torpedo* has large kidney-shaped electric organs toward the front of its flat body, one on each side of the eyes. With them it can deliver at least 220 volts, in jolt after jolt.

The electric ray *Torpedo*, like other rays and skates known to possess electric organs, behaves in a manner similar to that of the unrelated stargazers found along both Atlantic and Pacific coasts of southern North America. All of these marine fishes lie motionless on the bottom, waiting for prey to come along. With a sudden jolt of electricity they stun it as effectively as though they had produced an underwater explosion. Then the ray or skate or stargazer takes its time in devouring the stunned victim.

Other electric fishes are chiefly denizens of fresh waters, inhabiting particularly those so turbid that vision is of little use in finding food. In the Nile and other fresh waters of tropical Africa lives the electric catfish, whose body is surrounded by an electric organ like a sheath extending from the gill region to the base of the tail. Its discharge has been recorded to reach 350 volts. The Amazon, the Orinoco and other rivers of northeastern South America are home to the most powerful electric fish known: the eel-like *Electrophorus*. Captive six-foot individuals have driven the meter needle up to 550 volts, and produced enough current to make half a dozen 100-watt lamps flash like an electric sign.

Tribesmen in remote tributaries of these South American rivers are still using in a novel way the descendants of horses brought by the Spanish and Portuguese colonists. At fording places in rivers where electric eels are common, the native people tether a few horses on each bank. When someone wishes to cross the river, he first drives the horses through. He follows and catches the animals, promptly returning them to their tie ropes on the original bank. The electric eels discharge their batteries against the legs of the horses, and cannot reload their weapons before the fording party goes through unmolested.

The dreaded electric eel has its main electric organs along its flanks from well forward to its tail. As though these would not suffice, an additional, more slender electric organ extends along the lower surface for most of its length. Another is in the tail. All of these organs resemble those of other electric fishes in consisting of an orderly array of disk-shaped cells each contributing less than a seventh of a volt. An electric eel has from six thousand to ten thousand of these little generators in each of about seventy columns. Together they constitute about 40 per cent of the total bulk of the adult fish. When discharged simultaneously, they make the creature's head positive, its tail negative. Between these two, on all sides of the fish, an electric current flows through the water. It is this current that shocks anyone near by, and that the eel uses in stunning its prey. A corresponding current flows inside the electric eel, but vital organs such as its nervous system and swimming muscles seem to be electrically insulated by fatty tissue. Apparently this is why an electric eel does not electrocute itself or other electric eels.

Fishes able to produce large voltages employ their weapon in stunning animals as food. It would seem that they are not particularly discriminating, but rely primarily upon the fact that any appropriate victim will conduct electricity. They will swallow almost any object of the right general size, so long as it is a conductor. Electric eels have been found with pieces of iron in their stomachs.

Probably most of the fishes with electric organs too weak to produce a stunning shock use them only in navigation. At each pulse of their electrical charge, the body resembles a battery with one area positive, another negative. Through the water on all sides of its body the weak electric current flows in a pattern characteristic of the particular kind of fish. Such a pattern in the water is distorted by many different features of the environment. The earth's magnetic field distorts it slightly, and the form of the distortion changes according to the direction the fish is heading: north, south, west, east, up, down. A strong magnet hidden in the bottom mud is even more effective in altering the pattern, and gives the same differences according to the direction the fish heads.

Anything near a fish discharging pulses of electricity will affect the pattern if it conducts the current differently from the water touching the body of the fish. A layer of warmer or cooler water close by can do this. If a fish were sensitive enough to detect small changes in the areas from which its electric pulses leave and re-enter the body, it could learn a great deal about its surroundings.

Some of the eel-like electric fishes from the Nile River can be trained to respond to the stationary field of a hidden fixed magnet, showing that they are indeed alert to such features of their watery world. These fishes are also able to locate and distinguish among objects hung in an aquarium, according to whether they are good conductors (such as pieces of metal or chunks of meat) or non-conductors (such as blocks of plastic or ceramic materials). Usually they use this ability in avoiding any obstacle distorting the pattern of their electrical field.

Fishes with these special abilities are astonishingly sensitive. They will react to an electric current flowing past them when it is extremely slight (a gradient as little as 0.000,075 volt per inch). So refined a detection system would almost certainly respond to the presence of another fish. It could turn out to be the means, so long sought in vain, that permits herrings and other gregarious fishes to travel in close formation through the night. If each fish uses its electrical sensitivity to maintain awareness of its position in relation to others of the school, the group could wheel and dive in close formation without relying upon light or sound. This would be a three-dimensional equivalent of man-made radar, and represent a gain for fishes unmatched among land animals. Birds that migrate through the night are solitary fliers, unable without more light to maintain the flock pattern they would show by day.

With its high sensitivity to changes in the pattern of its own pulsed electrical field in the surrounding water, a fish may be able to make use also of the earth's fixed magnetic field. It is tempting to wonder whether a salmon, far out in the Pacific Ocean, relies upon an electromagnetic compass of this kind in directing its homing course toward the American river in which it hatched.

A few years ago, scientists would have been extremely reluctant to suggest a response by any animal to the earth's magnetic field. But currently the idea has acquired fresh appeal. Dr. Frank A. Brown, Jr., of Northwestern University recently presented statistical studies interpreted as proving that the common mud snail *Nassarius* does detect fixed magnetic fields. Both the earth's magnetic field and an artificial field ten times as strong were effective as guides for snails moving about in the water.

We tend to believe that what a snail can do a vertebrate animal should be able to do better. But when both a snail and a vertebrate show an ability man lacks, we can begin to wonder whether it may be a still broader feature in the animal kingdom. We may suspect that a number of individual animals close to one another could use variations in electrical fields as a means of communication. They might vary the rate of pulsing, or alter the pattern of voltages developed in the surrounding water. Such a method, hitherto undreamed of, would work well only at close range because of the high electrical resistance of water. Yet this would be a gain rather than a disadvantage, for it would insure privacy. Could we call such a low-voltage message an electrical whisper? Then the shocking display of an electric eel, which stuns nearby fishes for dinner, would be an electrical shout!

Now the hunt is on for details, both in the anatomy of lampreys, fishes and snails, and in the uses to which they put underwater electric pulses. At the same time, engineers recognize a fresh challenge. Can they imitate the electricity-sensing systems of underwater animals, enlarged to the dimensions that might be useful to man? We can see that the principles of aerodynamics apply equally to a flying fish, a soaring albatross and an intercontinental jet airplane. Surely, on a grand scale, something of comparable importance will be developed for the underwater realm, using a counterpart of the electrical sensitivity man has found in other living things. It may come as a sudden breakthrough in submarine radio or radar. Or it could lead to an entirely new understanding of the sea world our ancestors left so many eons ago.

III

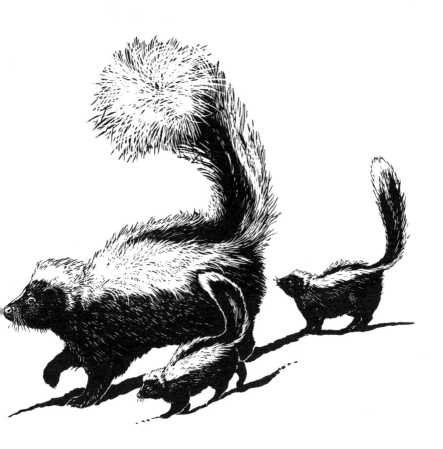

10. *The Importance of Odors*

NO ONE can guess confidently within a hundred million years when early forms of life began detecting molecules of distinctive chemical substances wafted to them in the seas of ancient times. This beginning long antedated the first eye and the earliest ear. It came eons prior to the day when animals began crawling out on land and testing the breeze for scents in air. The sense of smell is far older than the oldest hills. It preceded all other ways in which an animal can become aware of food, or a mate, or danger at a distance.

Despite its long history and man's own considerable

abilities in detecting and distinguishing among odors, the sense of smell remains mysterious. We gain little by comparing our relative odor-blindness to the perfume of female gypsy moths and the outstanding sensitivity of their mates. A gypsy moth shows no reaction to the aroma of hot biscuits, or pickles, or steak. Our nose is at least five times as sensitive to rosemary oil as the olfactory organs of a honeybee — but no more than a fortieth as able to detect methyl heptanone!

Each kind of animal has its own special odor spectrum. Generally it is most sensitive to compounds that have a significance under normal living conditions. The rabbit smells its way to a carrot or a dandelion. The cat or dog ignores these scents, but might find interest in the rabbit's trail. The scavenging dog sniffs vigorously at manure a cat disdains, but passes by the flowers and foliage a cat often takes time to brush against and smell appreciatively.

Our own sense of smell is restricted to a pair of grooves high in the nasal passages, where cells linked closely to the lower, forward portion of the brain are protected from the air passing them and kept clean by a thin film of flowing mucus. The area sensitive to odors totals less than the surface of a dime, and depends for its action upon about 600,000 special cells connected to our olfactory centers. Yet, with this meager and seemingly simple surface, we can learn to identify an apparently limitless number of odors.

To to be detected, a substance must first dissolve in the watery mucous film. Then, as it passes close to the ends of the sensory cells, it must be captured and held for a fraction of a second, perhaps linked to fat molecules in the cells' boundary layer. The amount that dissolves, however, may be incredibly small. If we pick up two pieces of milky quartz among the stones on a beach and strike one against the other in the dark our nose will detect a slightly sulfurous odor almost immediately after our eyes have caught the triboluminescent flash from molecules of rock jarred into emission of light. By day the flash is invisible, but the odor comes through. A few dust-sized particles of the rock have been freed by the impact, and found their way to the olfactory cells. But until that moment, the dust had been the water-scoured surface of a stone with the same chemical nature as glass! We don't expect any appreciable amount of quartz (or glass) to dissolve in water, or mucus, or fat. Yet enough goes into solution to alert us to a recognizable odor.

Among the substances to which our nose is most sensitive is musk, from the anal scent glands of the male musk deer, a small and much-persecuted mountain animal once common but now rare from Korea to the Himalayas. Musk, or its modern synthetic substitute, is diluted enormously and then used as a base for many perfumes. Even when too faint to be detected itself, it serves as a vehicle for more delicate fragrances, and continues to release them over a long time.

Chemists have calculated that any small area of diluted musk freeing 800,000 molecules per second will yield enough in two seconds to alert a human nose, and to let an expert positively identify the compound. At this rate, the active ingredient of crude musk spread in a thin film exposed to a continuous breeze would lose about one per cent of its potency in a million years.

A more familiar odor in North America is in a skunk's chemical armament. The active ingredient is ethanethiol (ethyl mercaptan), which is perceptible if as little as 0.000,000,000,000,071 ounce is inhaled. Such a trivial amount is still 19,400,000,000 molecules, which proves that our noses require about twelve thousand times as much skunk odor as musk to get the correct message to the brain.

Whenever anything we treasure becomes impregnated with ethanethiol, our chief concern is to find a way to eliminate the odor as quickly as possible. The old recipe for ridding garments of skunk scent was to bury them loosely in damp soil and let the earth absorb the aroma. A more reliable modern technique is to force air past the skunked cloth and into an activated charcoal filter similar to those used for removing kitchen odors. The enormous internal surfaces of the charcoal adsorb the smelly materials. Perhaps the surfaces of soil particles can act in the same way on buried objects.

Elimination of odors is important to animals too, as a protection from predators that hunt by scent. It may be

that quail and other ground-nesting birds gain concealment from enemies by letting body odors be absorbed into
the soil upon which the eggs are laid. Apparently these
birds hold tight together all feathers exposed to the passing
breeze while fluffing out those around the eggs or toward
the soil. If this interpretation is correct, then the lack of a
lining in the nest — a common feature — would actually
be an advantage and not an indication that the bird was
casual about its nest construction. Without a lining, the
bird would gain through fuller utilization of the odor-
absorbing power of the earth.

Concealment of odors is a truly complex problem, since
even the supposedly insensitive human nose is often critical
in discriminating and identifying scents. Not long ago an
entrepreneur began marketing a green solution as an odor
killer, claiming wonders for the "well-known deodorant"
powers of chlorophyll — to the surprise of scientists. Prior
to this, housewives often sought to confuse the nose of
visitors by adding to the household aroma from cooked
cabbage or fish the not unpleasant smell from the smolder-
ing end of a piece of cotton string hung over a doorknob.
Others burned a little incense, composed of exotic resins
and elemi—usually from the Orient—formed into cones
and slender wands supported on fibers of bamboo. Perhaps
incense itself was invented as a means for distracting wor-
shipers from other odors in pagan temples.

A very different method serves in the sea to stop a
predator from following an odor trail. The octopuses,
squids and cuttlefishes rely upon the anesthetic action of
an inky secretion they discharge when frightened. Until
recently this material was assumed to be merely an underwater smoke screen. Now it is known to be a chemical fog
dulling the olfactory organs of the morays and other fishes
that pursue these jet-propelled mollusks. No terrestrial or
freshwater animal is armed in a comparable way. Nor has
man discovered harmless anesthetics he might use to cover
up odors by reducing the sensitivity of human noses.

We are more likely to look for chemical means for repelling animals we don't want near us. Co-operative
projects are under way along the coasts of the Indian Ocean,
as well as of the Atlantic and Pacific, to discover substances

that will repel sharks. Most sharks come into surface waters close to shore only at night, when few swimmers are within reach. The number of people attacked annually by these scent-following creatures has never been large. Awareness of the danger has increased recently, however, now that so many people are venturing into deeper water or farther out. By donning rubber fins and either a simple snorkel or a tank of compressed gas to free themselves from frequent tripping to the surface, the frogmen invade the sharks' domain. The swimmer's peace of mind would be increased by carrying a chemical charm for instant release—something that would reliably drive any shark away.

A suitable substance for repelling sharks may yet be extracted from the skin of these predators. Certainly minnows and other fishes respond quickly to the dissolved odor from one of their kind that has been badly bruised or cut. Some compound from the skin warns the survivors to leave promptly. Even the odor of human skin repels most fishes, whereas it often seems to attract predatory sharks.

Hunters as well as fishermen are usually aware that human odors will frighten away the animal life they seek. A hunter needs to stalk his quarry in an upwind direction to prevent his scent from reaching it. The rest of us rarely realize that, while on a picnic or a walk through the fields and woodlands, our body scent carries across the landscape and causes hundreds of animals to dive into burrows or rush off terror-stricken. The late Roy Bedichek, one of Texas' outstanding naturalists, felt embarrassed that his "body was polluting the atmosphere on so vast a scale. There seemed something immoral about it. . . ."

Occasionally, we need the wind in our own direction to insure personal safety. We'll not forget the admonitions in advance nor the extreme caution with which a game warden and a native guide led us through the tick-infested dry grass up a low hill to a vantage point where we could watch a small herd of black rhinoceroses in South Africa. Not for a minute did the men take their eyes from the three-ton animals upwind and downslope from us.

The guide's special duty was to keep a continuous check on the breeze. If it changed direction, we must move swiftly. If the air movement ceased, we must leave at once. From experience the men knew how soon human scent could waft toward the monsters munching peacefully on thorn scrub two hundred yards away. They knew too how promptly black rhinos charge, and how little time we would have to race for the get-away car parked behind us far down the hill.

Sometimes an animal's sense of smell and dislike for the human odor can be used for man's protection. Often without knowing any reason for their action, cowhands of Texas and other parts of our Western states commonly follow an old precept. Each man at nightfall lays his lariat on the ground in a circle around his bedroll as a fence against rattlesnakes that might visit him and strike in darkness. Rattlers actually are repelled by human odor and are reluctant to cross a rope reeking of sweaty palms. Skunk scent and other odorous materials are even more effective in repelling snakes, but most of them offend human olfactory sense as well.

Some people seem able to turn the olfactory tables on the snake, by recognizing the odor of an undisturbed reptile and tracing it to its source. With practice a person can develop many olfactory skills of this kind. Helen Keller, who has been so successful at minimizing the handicaps of sightlessness, finds that she can associate a personal odor with many of the friends and visitors she meets, and that recall is as good for the olfactory feature as most people develop for a voice.

Manufacturers of toiletries might lead us to believe that body odors are uniformly unpleasant, undesirable and avoidable through use of their products. These generalizations are much too sweeping; they are overstatements aimed solely at increasing sales. Without being aware of it, most of us associate with the people we love best a skin fragrance that comes from no cream or soap or lotion. When a spouse goes away for a few days, the partner left behind may even find a little comfort from loneliness by nosing into a clothes closet in which the absent one's worn garments are hanging.

Usually we credit dogs with a special ability in distinguishing the scent of each human being. Certainly these

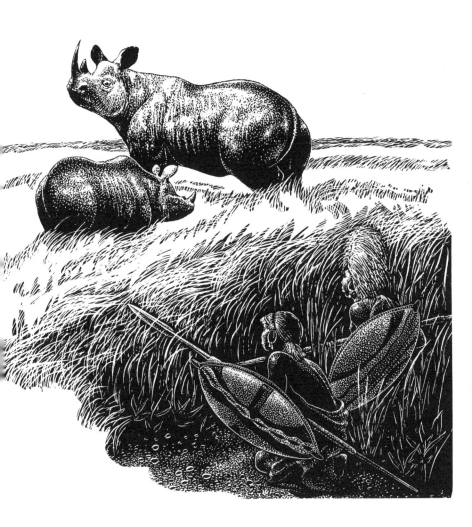

animals rely upon their noses far more than we. Many of them actually can identify the characteristic odor of a particular man or woman in a single footprint or a drop of saliva, even when the unknown individual has been encountered only through a glove or cap or scarf. The dog's nose may be confused by the trails of identical human twins, and still select one twin as the correct person to match an olfactory clue when the twins are encountered simultaneously.

So alert is the dog's olfactory sense that, if the animal is blindfolded, it can still point its nose straight at a rabbit. One experimenter described an "olfactory nystagmus" in a blindfolded dog before which a succession of caged rabbits passed on a rotating platform, like the imitation horses on a carousel. While following each rabbit in turn, the dog moved its head much as we shift our eyes in reading one line of print after another.

Few demonstrations of the importance of odors to a dog are more convincing than an animal of this kind standing outside a library or other public building, sniffing at each person who emerges while waiting for the one with the correct odor to come along. For a male dog, only the lure of a bitch in heat has higher priority than the master's scent. A professional burglar made a name for himself in scientific circles by taking advantage of this fact. Before going out in the night to rob a house guarded by a dog, the burglar played rough games with his pet bitch and got his clothes well impregnated with her odor. Even female watchdogs were usually so entranced by his doggy smell that they overlooked the strangeness of his human scent.

When a dog is separated from its accustomed human companion, it often acts as though unhappy. Sometimes this is due partly to being confined in a cage or pen at a boarding kennel and partly to a lack of other distractions. In her published volume of correspondence with George Bernard Shaw, the famous actress Mrs. Patrick Campbell tells of an Irishwoman who landed with her dog at an English port, only to learn that the animal would have to be held in quarantine. When the officials took the dog and put it in a basket, the woman slipped off her shoe and put it in the basket too. She knew that her pet would grieve less at the separation if it had the consolation of something with her odor, and was willing to limp to the train and the nearest shoe store to comfort the dog while complying with the law.

For dogs that hunt with muzzle to the ground, the world is rich in smells, sometimes to the point where objects in plain sight are overlooked. Even while asleep, these animals often produce little sounds and make slight movements as though dreaming of an exciting expedition through the underbrush. The dog's nose twitches and inhales breath in short, sharp gusts, just as the animal would do if awake and following a tantalizing trail.

Our odor spectrum may be much less colorful than that of many dogs. Certainly our language for describing scents is almost destitute. Usually we are forced to say that a substance smells somewhat like another, although we realize fully that they differ—in ways we cannot describe. In the middle of the eighteenth century, the Swedish naturalist Carolus Linnaeus attempted to remedy this deficiency by offering a system for describing odors, to be used as an aid in classifying plants.

Not until 1916 was any serious attempt made to replace the Linnaean system with a better one. Then the German psychologist H. Henning suggested that each odor might be assigned a place in a triangular prism whose corners were the scent qualities flowery, fruity, resinous, burnt, putrid and spicy. The idea was intriguing, but proved difficult to apply. Nine years later, the French physiologist H. Zwaardemaker offered an alternative with nine qualities: alliaceous (onions, garlic), ambrosiac (musk), aromatic (spices, burnt, including creosote), ethereal (fruits, wines), foul (bedbugs, French marigolds), fragrant (flowers), goaty (including rancid fats) and nauseous (decaying meat and feces). When this met with no wide acceptance, a simpler version was suggested in 1945, with merely four fundamental aspects on each of which a human nose might help assign a numerical value between 0 and 8: acid, burnt, fragrant and goaty. Perhaps no workable method will ever be devised, based upon the way people are affected by odorous materials.

Despite this failure to find an acceptable classification

for odors, we do recognize a considerable variety encountered in everyday life. Sir Arthur Conan Doyle had his character Sherlock Holmes state that identification of seventy-five different scents was essential to good detective work—without listing them. The modern Japanese go farther, enjoying a parlor game in which objects carrying some one of two hundred standardized odors are passed around and the participants asked to name the substance. Success in a game of this kind requires both a good nose and an olfactory education.

One surprising feature is that some people are unaware of certain scents. In every thousand one or two detect no odor in the skunk's arsenal. A few more find it fragrant, when strong enough to stimulate their olfactory sense—and drive everyone else away! A great many scents, in fact, change their apparent nature when concentrated. A very little musk is as fragrant as any flower; a powerful whiff of it is nauseating. Nor are we unusual in this. Many insects, such as the carrion-loving bluebottle fly, are attracted to a mixture of certain chemicals in air over a tenfold range of concentration. But with further increase they are repelled.

Sensitivity to specific odors may be inherited in varying degrees. Most albino people are handicapped by relative insensitivity to the whole spectrum of scents. Not only do they lack coloring in hair, skin and iris of the eyes, but their olfactory areas have none of the yellow pigment other human beings possess. It is tempting to wonder whether the pigment has anything to do with smell. Yet biochemists do not mention pigments when they suggest that odorous substances are ones that play a tune in the nose through differential inactivation of eight different enzymes in the boundaries of the olfactory cells.

Those of us with able noses can train them to discriminate among a surprising number of scents. Most of these odors are particularly effective at stimulating our memory to recall previous encounters with the same fragrance. A faint whiff of sea air, no matter whether it carries enough salt dust to swirl through the nasal passages and reach the salt-taste centers on the forward and side edges of the tongue or contains molecules from decaying seaweeds in storm drift, gives a fresh lift to the human spirit and recalls crashing waves, hovering gulls, and perhaps a hip-booted fisherman casting in the surf. A person's eyes need not be open when, as he tops a rise on a western road, the breeze brings the spicy scent of sagebrush, for the mind to picture the rolling hills covered by green-gray shrubs whose leaves and stems seem crisp in the noonday sun. Even the fragrance of lilac perfume from a bottle is enough to flood the mind with a memory of tall bushes wearing a springtime green on smooth foliage below purple flowers visited by yellow-and-black tiger swallowtail butterflies.

Attempts to increase sales by adding scents to merchandise are spreading. Makers of plastic flowers coat their products with a compound said to release a flowerlike fragrance for four months. Plastic bags scented with cedarwood are used to combine nose appeal with dustproofing of blankets. The day may not be distant when a transparent envelope containing oranges in the grocery store will smell of oranges, and mouse traps come redolent of bacon to lead victims to the final meal of cheese. Publishers are testing the effect of adding a saddle-leather scent to western novels, and a yeasty fresh-bread smell to cookbooks. Envelope makers add wintergreen or peppermint flavor to the adhesive licked to seal in a letter, giving the sender a chance to swirl the scent molecules through the throat to the nose, where the odor will be detected and enjoyed. Movie showmen have already tried wafting scents past the viewers' seats, to increase the illusion of reality. The "smellies" can furnish a pine-woods atmosphere, the pungent aroma of burning leaves, the combined fragrances of a flower garden, or the atmosphere of a pub to match the mood the picture is intended to induce.

Our noses grow accustomed to an odor if the amount available remains the same for many minutes or increases very slowly. Coal miners have overcome this handicap by taking caged canaries into the tunnels with them. These birds can smell nothing, but they collapse from poisonous coal gas before the concentration becomes fatal to the workers. So long as the canaries remain alert, the men need not fear asphyxiation.

To some extent we overcome this characteristic of the

olfactory cells by sampling the air a sniff at a time. Sniffing creates a turbulence in the nasal passages. It brings more of the incoming air close to the sensory centers, rather than letting it pass by at lower levels in the nose. Sometimes an isolated sniff lets us identify a new odor, for the nose which has grown accustomed to one scent is still as alert as ever to a different fragrance. As the components in a mixed perfume vary in concentration with time, an expert can become aware of one after another until every kind present has been identified correctly.

Even under the best conditions, we are not always alert to odors in the air we inhale. As recently as 1950 a regular fluctuation was discovered in our ability to detect substances by smell. All normal people become more sensitive to aromas reaching their nose in late morning and again in late afternoon. Sensitivity falls off markedly soon after lunch. But if the noon meal is omitted, our interest in all fragrances maintains its late-morning level. Our state of nutrition, which can be measured by checking the blood-sugar concentration, is a real factor determining how much information we get from our nose. Is this the reason that a fresh cup of coffee tastes so good before breakfast, or the explanation for our alertness to odors when we go for a walk outdoors at dawn? How many olfactory sensations are important enough to us that we would willingly do without a meal to enjoy them to the full?

Olfactory sensitivity differs too according to sex. Women detect the odor from a mixture consisting of equal parts of the fatty substance cholesterol with testosterone acetate (a derivative of the male sex hormone) at lower concentrations than men can. Children, men and women beyond reproductive age report little or no odor from exaltolide, a substance with fifteen carbon atoms per molecule and a chemical constitution similar to that of the civet used by perfumers. Apparently the sex hormone estrogen circulating in the blood is necessary to let a person find fragrance in exaltolide. Women in their reproductive years, especially for a week or two following each monthly period, prove to have good sensitivity for the substance. If men are given an injection of estrogen, they too can smell the material.

Probably our sex hormones affect the sense of smell to

an extent far greater than is realized even by scientists. White rats show this in relation to the odor of eucalyptus. Males are sensitive to eucalyptus only if they have normal amounts of testosterone; castrated ones detect none of the spicy smell we do. Female white rats, however, are much more aware of eucalyptus after they have been desexed, and hence lack estrogen in the blood. Strangely enough, female white rats seem unable to distinguish the sex of other rats by smell, whereas a normal mature male white rat shows a truly remarkable discrimination among juvenile and mature males, females not in heat, females in heat, desexed females, and desexed females receiving estrogen treatment.

The most famous example of sex differences in detection of odors was discovered by the patient French naturalist J. Henri Fabre while watching Chinese silkworm moths. Females of this insect are completely insensitive to the scent lure with which they summon mates. Yet marked males of the silkworm moth have been known to fly upwind seven miles to a fragrant female of their kind. For years this ability of the males has been quoted as outstanding, perhaps without serious competition elsewhere in the animal kingdom.

The chemical compound with which a female silkworm moth attracts mates is highly specific; no other species seem aware of it. In 1959, the Nobel laureate Adolph Butenandt of the Max Planck Institute for Biochemistry in Munich succeeded in analyzing it. He found it to be an alcohol with sixteen carbon atoms per molecule, a yellowish greasy material from which the human nose gains only a slight, pleasant odor suggesting that of leather. In the following year, a research team working for the United States Agricultural Service at Beltsville, Maryland, extracted a similar compound, with eighteen carbon atoms per molecule, from females of the European gypsy moth, which has become such a pest since its introduction into America in 1868. The Beltsville chemists also synthesized the substance, and found that male moths could detect it in quantities as little as 0.000,000,000,000,004 ounce— about 200,000 molecules. This level of sensitivity is only about eight times as great as ours is to musk.

The odor of the male has meaning for many animals, and may have more significance in mankind than we realize. Its most astonishing effects have been discovered among laboratory mice. Female mice show adjustments of their sexual cycle when they detect the odor of males of their own species. In addition, as was learned during 1960 at the National Institute for Medical Research in London, England, recently mated female mice will fail to become pregnant if they are subjected to the smell of strange males. Under crowded conditions they cannot be on sniffing terms with all mice in the colony. Under these circumstances, most of them fail to bear young. A similar response under wild conditions or in the human species would soon relieve overpopulation.

A characteristic odor that corresponds to a whole species of animal is much easier for our nose to recognize. We know one scent as that of dog, another as that of horse —without regard for breed. An ammoniacal odor in a warehouse or other building can alert us to mice. In the aquatic world, minnows can be taught to distinguish among their own and various other species merely from water that has flowed past the unseen fishes. Sometimes man, who admits to an olfactory sense less reliable than that in other animals, claims to be able to distinguish one human race from another by smell. "Fee, Fie, Fo, Fum, I smell the blood of an Englishman."

Occasionally a racial or tribal odor is real, although acquired and not inborn. To the American Indians, the white settlers stank—and this may have been true when a bath was a Saturday-night event. But these complaints ceased when the Indians began to wear clothes and adopt the white man's other habits. The Navajo Indians, who live in hogans on the big reservations in Arizona and New Mexico, have a distinctive odor that sometimes can be detected many yards away. It is from the wood smoke produced inside the ill-ventilated house, and a fragrance that is quickly acquired by any white man who goes to live in a Navajo's hogan. Similarly, the odor we find unpleasant when close to many of Africa's native people in their home territory proves to be rancid fats, particularly butter, with which they smear their bodies to repel insects.

Putrefaction of butter produced butyric acid, a substance to which our nose is particularly sensitive.

A home odor is very important to honeybees. Each worker leaving the hive for field duties carries a sample of this fragrance locked in a special scent sac. As she returns and alights on the sill at the hive entrance, she opens the sac as though displaying a pass badge to the guardians of the portal. Only bees with the proper hive odor are admitted. The odor itself is a wonderful mixture of scents from all the different flower products stored in the hive, and is distinctive only because each hive contains a unique sample of the nectars, pollens and resins available in the area. If workers from two hives are allowed to feed for a few weeks from only two or three food sources, the hive odors become indistinguishable. If the two hives are interchanged, the bees notice no significant difference. Field bees then return to whichever hive is in the correct geographical location.

Like beehives, our houses acquire unique odors which a person with a sensitive nose detects when entering the door. We tend to like the aroma of home, and notice when its nonspecific average is accented by coffee or fresh paint, by laundry drying or yeast bread rising, by turkey roasting or carrots burning. Our parents' homes have special attraction too, whether the dominant fragrance is of plants in bloom or repolished brassware, a particular blend of pipe tobacco or something on the kitchen stove—cookies or home-made pickles or the soup pot.

When we leave the house, city odors may assail us. In self-protection we may prefer to ignore messages the nose sends brainward. Or, with modern means of transportation, we flit from city to city by airplane high above the ground, missing the piny fragrance of Maine, the citrus fragrance of Florida or California, the spicy scent of western chaparral under the summer sun. In a plane we are above where even the birds fly, and need our nose still less than they.

Will a continuation or extension of aerial travel make us more like birds? These feathered fliers are notoriously sharp of eye, keen of hearing, but unaware of odors. The nostrils high in the beak still admit air, which needs to be cleaned of dust, to be adjusted in temperature and humidity before reaching the lungs. The beak, moreover, is used in managing food and preening feathers. This feature on a bird's head plays too many roles to disappear along with the sense of smell.

But what of the human nose? Already in many places air-conditioning equipment removes the dust, adjusts the temperature and humidity into the most desirable range. Contact lenses eliminate the value of a nose in supporting eyeglasses. If we cease to educate our noses, will we not miss fragrances of importance? Would the nose disappear altogether?

How much will olfaction, which is currently our most neglected sense, mean to mankind a thousand or ten thousand years from now? Will anyone then know the scent of apple blossoms in the spring, of roses and wisteria in the summer, of witch hazel as the last of autumn's flowers? Or discover Australia as a continent and a country with a national odor—of eucalyptus?

Fortunately, the future of the human nose does not depend alone on its ability to condition air and to distinguish the fragrance of a flower from the aroma of a skunk. We send countless odors to our olfactory tracts by the back doorway, from the throat, and depend upon our sense of smell in savoring the foods we eat. Without the mysterious nasal sense our meals would be dull indeed—as though we had a perpetual head cold. So long as we continue to get our nourishment in the conventional way, rather than as pills to be swallowed untasted, the human nose—of whatever size or shape—is here to stay.

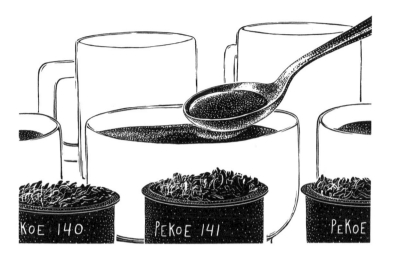

KOE 140   PEKOE 141   PEKOE

11. *The Limits of Taste*

FINE FOODS are distinguished by their flavors, and each nation prides itself on particular traditions. What would French or Italian cooking be without onions and garlic? How would we know the special dishes of Mexico and southward if not for chili powder made from hot red peppers? Where would a Far Eastern cook turn for seasonings if her shelf was bare of ginger from tropical Asia and cardamon—for curries—from Ceylon? For that matter, how would we like our prime steaks innocent of salt and true pepper from the East Indies?

Today's signs advertise "28 Flavors" appealing to our tastes, or invite us to sample meals given such artful seasoning as to make them irresistible. Even the plainest food gains zest through addition of condiments in judicious touches. Restaurateurs take advantage of this fact, and make available to their patrons an assortment that has become almost standardized: sugar, salt, pepper, vinegar,

135

mustard, tomato sauce and perhaps tabasco or spicy Worcestershire.

Ingredients for modern seasoning of food come from all over the world, and from the realm of chemistry as well. So smoothly does this commerce operate today that it is easy to forget its evolution since the times of swashbuckling buccaneers and the spice trade that preceded colonialism. To get spices overland more reliably, Marco Polo journeyed all the way from Venice to the court of Kublai Khan and back—to jail. The flavors of the Orient beckoned Christopher Columbus westward across the Atlantic four times, always seeking a sea lane to China and the East Indies. When Vasco da Gama led the Portuguese around the southern tip of Africa, it was in search of a better route to the islands of the Indian Ocean: to Ceylon for cinnamon and cardamon, to Zanzibar and Madagascar for cloves and to other ports for almonds and ginger and pepper. Only later did the spice trade become the prerogative of the Dutch and the English.

So great a demand for substances appealing to taste could not be satisfied indefinitely through a monopoly. Gradually the plants from which spices came were smuggled into other parts of the world and grown there too. But out of these changes in commerce came a new internationalism. Now a department store advertises honey from almost every part of the globe, and the judging of teas, coffees and wines has become a business mixed with art, requiring "tea tasters," "coffee tasters" and "wine tasters" who are specialists at blending or classifying.

A professional taster swallows none of the material he samples. He takes a small sip and lets his tongue explore. At the same time any odorous components rise through his throat into his nose, and he savors them as well. His interest is in the complete effect, not in separating those sensations received through his tongue from those reaching him in other ways. Actually, it is almost impossible to separate taste from odor while testing any but the simplest foods. Our real distinctions among flavors are olfactory, rather than through taste. If the nose is blocked, we cannot tell a piece of apple placed on the tongue from a piece of raw potato. Both are faintly sweet, but no more than that.

All of us judge foods also through a delicate awareness in the realm of touch, distributed widely over lips, gums, tongue and palate. This helps us learn of texture, and also to recognize astringent materials which compete for moisture in the mouth. Chokecherries and unripe persimmons "pucker up" the lining of the mouth, even retarding the flow of saliva. The chemical "heat" of mustard or chili peppers, like the tang of "nippy" cheese, appeals to these senses that are neither taste nor smell.

Of all the condiments we add at the table, only salt, sugar and vinegar actually appeal to taste. Salty, sweet, sour and bitter are the sole taste sensations we can appreciate. And bitter is a flavor we come to enjoy only through experience. Bitter things are often poisonous, and our inborn distrust of them must stem from far back in the evolution of mankind. A few people manage to go through life without meeting a single bitter taste. Others develop a liking for the bitterness beer gains from hops, or the bitter flavor of vermouth wine, which comes from the addition of herb extracts such as gentian, quinine and wormwood.

To trigger one or more of these taste sensations for an adult person, a substance must reach the taste buds borne by the tip, the edges and the back part of the upper surface of the tongue. We have about ten thousand of them altogether. Those responding to sweet substances are chiefly at the tip. Salty sensations come from all around the sides and tip of the tongue, whereas sour is largely restricted to the sides. Bitter is located well back on the upper surface. A drop of Epsom-salt solution tastes salty if applied to the tip or edges of the tongue, and bitter when it reaches the area far back.

Each taste bud is a little goblet-shaped cluster of cells, and measures about 1/360 of an inch across. Children have taste buds studding the hard palate, soft palate, walls of the throat and the central upper surface of the tongue as well. By maturity, however, we lose them over all of these areas. As we age, many of the remaining ones disappear too. Our sense of taste fades at a comparable rate, and we are likely to put more sugar in our coffee. Young adults can identify a sugar solution as being sweet at a third the concentration required to give a taste to an elderly person.

Rarely can we taste anything at a distance. Taste is a contact sense, depending upon molecules of the flavorful substance dissolved in saliva on the tongue. Human saliva is more than water, however. It is faintly acid and contains a number of buffering agents that tend to neutralize anything more acid or alkaline in the mouth. It seems also to be a particularly personal secretion, as unique perhaps as our fingerprint patterns. Some compounds can be tasted only when dissolved in our own saliva. If dissolved in water or in the saliva of another person, they remain flavorless even when placed on a suitably sensitive area of the tongue that has been washed and dried carefully. Yet taste appears suddenly if a drop of our own saliva is added to the mixture.

By comparison with the sensitivity of the human nose to odors, our taste buds seem crude. To induce a taste sensation we need at least twenty-five thousand times as many molecules as to alert the olfactory sense. Bitterness, moreover, is detected at concentrations a thousand times less than those required if a sweet, sour or salty substance is to be identified. Probably it is a warning—the last possible one—against swallowing poisonous substances.

The operation of taste buds would be far easier to understand if the chemists could show that particular kinds or shapes of molecules correspond to the four different taste sensations we experience. Sourness is the only one that matches a single chemical agent. This taste is induced by atoms of hydrogen bearing a positive electrical charge— the hydrogen ions that give acids of all kinds their distinctive nature. Solutions with equal concentrations of hydrogen ion are equally sour, and indistinguishable from one another if interactions with saliva and cues from odor are eliminated.

"Salty" is a much more mysterious quality. It too comes from ions, such as the sodium ions and chloride ions formed when table salt (sodium chloride) dissociates in water. Both the positively charged sodium ions and the negatively charged chloride ions contribute toward the saltiness we detect, but each of these ions is merely the most effective member of a whole series. All members of both series induce a salty flavor, although they differ slightly in ways we cannot describe unless they stimulate the bitter sense as well. The other "salty" positive ions are potassium, lithium, ammonium and magnesium. The "salty" negative ions, in addition to chloride, are bromide, iodide, fluoride, nitrate, sulfate, carbonate and tartrate. Almost any combination of these two series, such as sodium tartrate or ammonium chloride will free ions into water and give us a salty sensation.

A great many animals, from guinea pigs to honeybees, show that their taste centers cannot distinguish among the positive and negative ions that give us a salty taste. If these animals are kept on a diet lacking in a normal amount of salt, they develop a craving for it. Under such circumstances they will eagerly take any solution we find to be salty. At the same time they show no abnormal interest in those we find sour, sweet or bitter.

For animals that feed solely on plants, salt hunger can be very real. They develop it because of a great difference in the proportions of sodium and potassium in vegetation and flesh. The plants they eat are rich in potassium, poor in sodium. A very little potassium satisfies an animal's needs, but sodium is necessary in quantity for growth. To convert vegetation into meat, a herbivorous creature has to salvage all of the sodium it can while disposing of the excess potassium. If it loses additional sodium salts in sweat, a serious deficiency in sodium is likely to develop. The symptoms are muscle cramps and weakness, just as they are in people who sweat profusely without taking salt tablets.

If given an opportunity, a herbivorous animal suffering from salt hunger will show that its taste buds distinguish sodium salts from all others in a way we cannot match. To us, sodium chloride in reasonable amounts is almost indistinguishable from potassium chloride, whereas the taste of sodium carbonate (washing soda) or sodium bicarbonate (baking soda) is quite different. The herbivorous animal is not fooled. In the wild it will make tremendous migrations to places where the soil contains large amounts of sodium salt—any sodium salt that gives us a salty taste. It will not patronize a place with chlorides of potassium, ammonium, magnesium or lithium, although these seem so similar to our tongues.

The farmer who puts out a salt block for his domestic animals is saving them from salt deficiency and the urge to travel to a salt lick. Deer, antelope and other cud chewers are easily baited within sight by offering salt where they can reach it. Gigantic giraffes and other African game animals travel for many miles to a famous salt lick beside a dirt road through the Royal Game Park just outside the city of Nairobi in Kenya. The giraffes stand there for hours every day, until they are satisfied that no lion will attack them while they stiffly spread their forelegs wide and let themselves down into an awkward position in which they can lick the ground.

Our own sensation of saltiness is undistinguished, but we do use expressions in speech that link salty to sweet tastes. We talk of one lake as having "sweet water" and another as being a "salt lake," even if it is alkaline with carbonates of sodium or potassium rather than charged with sodium chloride. Somewhere in our tongues the salty taste must be linked to sweet, although how this occurs is still unknown. If we put on one side of our tongue a solution of sodium chloride just too dilute to be identified as salty, and then apply something sweet to the opposite side, we suddenly taste the salt too. The converse is true as well. Interactions of this type seem to account for our realization that we can "bring out the flavor" by adding a little salt to a sweet melon, or by using a sweet pickle with salty meat. The sweetness of ice cream is enhanced by a few salty nuts in it, and the salt of a cracker is more striking after a bit of jelly is added.

In our minds we often equate "sweet" with "good," and assume that a sweet-tasting substance will be safe to eat. Yet our taste buds are ready to mislead us. We get a sweet taste from sodium chloride itself if the solution is very weak (around eleven hundredths of one per cent) and an even more convincing sweet sensation from potassium chloride at roughly half this concentration. So many salts of beryllium have a sweet flavor that this material was originally called glucinum—the "sweet element." Some salts of lead are sweet to the tongue, but no less poisonous. Actually, the synthetic compound credited with being the sweetest substance known ("P-4000," which is an *n* propyl derivative of 4-alkoxy-3-amino-nitrobenzene) is so toxic that even the insignificant amounts of it needed to flavor foods are dangerous to use.

We also equate "sweet" with "sugar," and this is generally correct. There is good reason, however, for preferring the sugar from cane or beets as a flavoring for foods; this particular sugar (sucrose) affects our taste buds more than any other. By tasting solutions of different sugars at equal concentrations, we can arrange them in a series of progressively lessening sweetness: sucrose (saccharose), fructose (fruit sugar), maltose (malt sugar), glucose (grape sugar = dextrose), and lactose (milk sugar). Nor can any regularity be seen in this sequence. "Blood sugar" is a mixture of glucose and fructose, absorbed from the alimentary canal where they are produced by digestion. Makers of candy bars sometimes advertise that their products are rich in the "energy sugar" dextrose, which reaches the blood stream more quickly than sucrose because it needs no digestion. Saccharin and cyclamate (Sucaryl) give us a sweet taste, sometimes followed by a bitter aftertaste, but are nonnourishing because they are not digested or absorbed by the body.

When other animals confuse these same chemical compounds with sugar solutions, we conclude that a sweet taste is part of their sensory spectrum too—even if they lack taste buds or a true tongue. The front feet of blowflies and butterflies bear most of their sense organs for taste. If they can step into any solution we recognize as sweet, they readily distinguish it from salty, sour or bitter. A blowfly's front feet, in fact, are almost five times as sensitive to some sugars as its mouth. Starvation for ten days increases this sensitivity to sugars until it is as much as seven hundred times as acute as when the blowfly is well fed.

Many animals have a "sweet tooth." They are so eager for anything with a sweet taste that candy becomes an ideal reward. A horse or a dog, like a child, learns tricks far more quickly when good performance leads promptly to a piece of sugar. The cat, by contrast, shows no interest in sweets. Its taste buds send no messages to the brain when sugar solutions are spread on its tongue. This difference may well explain some of the cat's independent ways, and its seeming resistance to being taught tricks.

Mice and rats, on the other hand, behave much as a person does when working in a candy shop, with access to sweets of many kinds. At first they will choose the sweetest and eat to excess. Soon, however, they become satiated and, if a variety of sugar solutions having different concentrations remains available, the rodents take an occasional sample but show a preference for an intermediate strength—about ten per cent sucrose.

Mixtures of solutions we identify as sweet with others that are salty, sour or bitter seem to affect other animals in a comparable way. Like ourselves, honeybees are most sensitive to bitterness. Additions of quinine to attractive sugar solutions quickly repel all bees, flies and butterflies. For these creatures too the bitterest substances are among the most poisonous. They are alkaloids, such as strychnine, brucine, nicotine and quinine. Quinine has become a reference standard, because it is less toxic than the others. For popular comparisons, however, it may never replace bile as the basis for the phrase "bitter as gall." We've often wondered about this expression. Who goes around tasting gall, to know that it is bitter? Bile ("gall") is a complex mixture of compounds, several of which contribute toward its bitterness.

A bitter taste is obtained from many materials that are not alkaloids. A strong solution of potassium chloride is bitter as well as salty and slightly sour. Salicylic acid (aspirin) is bitter and dangerous only if taken in excess. Picric acid is intensely bitter and very poisonous. Iodides are bitter in addition to being salty. So are some positively-charged ions, such as magnesium from epsom salt, and silver from silver chloride—used frequently as an antiseptic in the eyes, from which it reaches the back of the tongue via the tear canals and nose.

Since the early 1930's, it has been clear that the ability to taste some substances is inherited. Thousands of pedigrees have now been followed for the organic compound phenylthiocarbamide (PTC), which can be synthesized inexpensively. About seventy people in every hundred recognize its bitterness at low concentrations. The other thirty are "non-tasters," who detect nothing in a solution until the concentration of PTC is about a thousand times higher than is needed to alert the majority. "Tasters" have inherited a dominant gene that confers upon them this curious ability.

Tasters and nontasters of PTC can be found among anthropoid apes too. Rats, however, uniformly reject solutions containing the compound—and for good reason. Even small doses of it are fatal to them if administered by stomach tube. When this was discovered, chemists set out to explore all related organic compounds and soon found one that was at least as toxic but had no flavor a rat could detect. Under the trade name Antu this poison is incorporated into a variety of foods to be left where unwanted rats will find them.

Comparable methods have seldom been applied to rendering bad-tasting medicines more palatable. Instead, the drug manufacturers have sought ways to get their pills past the taste buds without annoying the patient. Sugar-coating the pill is often enough, if it can be swallowed quickly. An old-fashioned gelatine capsule gives the medicine a tasteless covering that does not dissolve until it reaches the stomach. For compounds that might be regurgitated with unpleasant effects, the new enteric coatings are surer, for they remain in place through the stomach and into the intestine.

Despite these precautions, the taste (and often an odor as well) may be detected as soon as the compound is absorbed into the blood and is carried by that route to the tongue and nose. Similarly, an intravenous injection of vitamin B_4 in the forearm leads in about eight seconds to detection of its peanutlike flavor—as soon as blood carrying the material circulates to the mouth. Patients taking the arsenical Neosalvarsan by injection report tasting and smelling it after a similarly brief time. These sensations are not blocked by a head cold or by local anesthetics, but they disappear completely if the taste buds are impaired.

We have no reason to envy other animals a more complete sense of taste, although some of them can regulate their eating through quite different responses than we show to taste. The rabbit with its seventeen thousand taste buds and the cow with twenty-five thousand appear to detect neither more nor less than we do with our ten thousand. It would be a mistake, moreover, to conclude that a parrot enjoyed eating chili peppers at their fiery hottest because its mouth has only about four hundred taste buds. Parrots actually have more taste buds than other birds, many of which get along with from twenty to sixty. Any bird seems able to use its smaller number of sense centers in evaluating its food.

A recent count of taste buds on the tongues of individual domestic pigeons showed a range from twenty-seven to fifty-nine. Yet tame pigeons we used to keep often proved that they could detect starch as differing from protein. Probably gray squirrels can too, for whenever these animals found dry shelled corn we had put out for the pigeons while the birds were flying, the squirrels used their chisel teeth to cut out the white, glistening embryo from each kernel. After this protein-rich portion of the kernel had been removed by a squirrel, no pigeon would do more than lift, taste and discard the seed. With our larger number of taste buds we cannot distinguish between starch and protein in a corn kernel.

So far no one has discovered how our own taste centers operate, let alone why they find no sweetness in starch or glycogen as some other animals do. No one is sure, either, whether anything can be done to extend our sense of taste except by paying more attention to the messages our brain receives from the tongue. Scientists have largely ignored this sense, perhaps because it has no real defense or communication value. Smell, hearing and vision could all be called "get-away senses," for they can warn us of distant features in our surroundings. Taste is immediate.

With our limited repertoire of tastes, embellished by a reasonable variety of olfactory accents and subtle appreciations of texture, we decide with each mouthful of food whether to swallow or not. This is actually a decision of considerable finality for, after any morsel has been propelled past the last taste buds at the back of the tongue, it is on its way down.

The acceptability of a food is not, however, an attribute of the food. Instead, it is principally an expression of our culture, our food habits and the pressure of hunger. Many a person balks at eating cheeses or aged eggs which others consider delicious. In many parts of the world we need the curiosity and courage credited to members of the Explorers Club to sample a python filet, a whale steak, tentacles of octopus, or a piece of extinct mammoth taken from arctic soil that has been deep-frozen for fifteen thousand years. Only imminent starvation, however, seems adequate to most of us as grounds for condoning cannibalism.

The rules of good taste in food for man are as varied as tribal customs of other kinds. Hindus and other vegetarians fail to understand neighbors who eat fish and flesh. Moslems and Jews feel that their reasons for avoiding pork should be convincing. Yet, if we look into the old Hebraic rules on diet, we find that Moses authorized the children of Israel to eat locusts, grasshoppers and beetles (Leviticus II: 21-22).

African natives relish the grub stage of the world's largest beetle—*Megasoma goliathus.* Mexican markets offer fried grasshoppers and trays full of cooked caterpillars. In fact, a maguey caterpillar at the bottom of a cup of *tequila* is as much a mark of good taste as an olive in a martini. We have no reason to doubt that insects could tickle the palates of Anglo-Americans just as well as shrimp, lobster, oysters, snails or abalone steak. Insects might even cease to be so much of a problem for man if he took to eating those that now attack his crops. That we avoid these potential foods is no reflection on our taste buds. These sense organs are ready to savor any delicacy, if we are willing.

By disregarding taste and related senses in choosing our food, we sometimes fare less well than our fellow creatures in the wild. So long as they have the ingredients available, they select a reasonably balanced diet. In the wild we might do so too. Now, however, our civilized habits get in our way. They induce a surprising number of people to eat themselves into semi-starvation, through selection of nutritionally inadequate foods. Or we overeat. We even transfer a handicap to our house pets when we give them human food.

Unavoidably, our cultural taboos and emotional preferences in foods have a strong influence on our lives. Our bodies are composed almost exclusively of molecules from the foods we eat, and the variety is limited. Even if people had genetic heritages as nearly identical as those in a colony of inbred laboratory rats, their differences in food habits would go a long way toward producing individual, national and racial characteristics we would recognize. Our genetic heritage is only uniform enough for each human being to be politically equal to every other. But rare indeed are the people who are equal enough to be interchangeable. Dietary differences help keep them unlike.

To the degree that "we are what we eat," we can survey the meals on the tables of the world to learn where civilization is taking us. What we see will mirror economic state and the tastes to which people have grown accustomed. It will show also signs of change, rapid in the highly cultured areas and slow in the more primitive. Now that any place on earth is within a few days' travel of every other, and more people are exploring the tastes of distant lands, progress toward an international diet enjoyed worldwide seems inevitable. Where will it lead us? If flavors are to affect our future, at least there are no limits on taste!

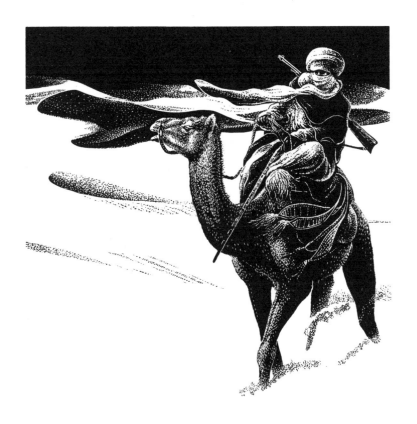

12. *The Mystery of Thirst*

SOMEHOW it seems fitting for one of the earliest mentions of thirst to come from the deserts of Egypt. About forty centuries ago, the henchman Sinuhe who served as administrator under King Amenemhet I, was felled by thirst as he crossed the Isthmus of Suez. In one of the treasured records of ancient Egypt is the story of his despair, with his tongue stuck to the roof of his mouth, his throat burning, his whole body demanding something to drink. "This," he told himself, "is the taste of death."

147

Today, these sensations are still a real hazard. No man can survive for three weeks if his water supply is cut off completely. With water he might last a month without food. Yet we appear to have a plentiful supply of water in our bodies: between 50 and 60 per cent of our adult weight. Our leeway is roughly a fifth of this amount. If we lose more, we die. If we lose less, we survive and can replenish our inner store. It makes no difference whether the loss is so sudden that it occurs in a single day, as sometimes happens to people lost in hot deserts, or comes over a period of weeks. In 1821 a prominent Frenchman committed suicide by persistently refusing to drink anything; he held out for seventeen days. On the fifteenth day, he might have saved himself. Castaways who have been fifteen days without water have survived the ordeal.

Most of us never come anywhere near such extremes of thirst. Yet all of us experience this sensation. Amazingly, we respond to its gentle urgings in the most casual ways and still manage to maintain our inner diffuse reserves of water with outstanding accuracy. From our hidden "water pool" we lose daily about two-thirds of a quart by perspiration and as moisture in the air we exhale. On a normal balanced diet, we discharge about a quart of water merely to flush out the waste products of each day's metabolism. At the same time, we gain about a third of a quart as "metabolic water" synthesized daily through the digestion of even dry foods. But without wet foods and liquids in our diet, we would quickly incur a serious deficit. Under the faint prodding of thirst, we make good the deficit almost automatically. Automatically, too, we compensate for extra losses or extra gains. How do we know when we've had enough? The sense of thirst is so vague that we are hard put to say just where we feel it.

Children soon learn that their fathers and mothers are reluctant to ignore a request for water. How many parents today do as ours did: order us to hold a little water in the mouth for a few minutes, to "let it quench our thirst" and incidentally keep us quiet? The notion that dryness of the mouth causes thirst goes back a long way, and was made respectable a few decades ago by the great endocrinologist Walter B. Cannon. Unfortunately, it is not an adequate explanation. Dryness which comes from nervousness, long-winded public speaking or breathing through the mouth during vigorous exercises, as well as from a reduced flow of saliva, can be relieved with a little lemon juice or a sour pickle that will stimulate the salivary reflex. These palliatives will not conceal true thirst for more than a few minutes.

We feel thirst so often when we are dehydrated, when our dehydration is leading to a reduction in the flow of saliva and a dryness of the mouth, that we condition ourselves into believing dryness and thirst to be synonymous. Actually, we can become desperately thirsty while our salivary glands, stomach, blood stream and bladder are all loaded with water. Deliberately or unconsciously, bartenders make use of this in selling their wares. They encourage thirst by putting out free dishes of salty, mouth-watering tidbits: pretzels, potato chips, popcorn, peanuts. Saliva flows freely. Yet the back of the throat reports that it is parched. How about another drink? The parching is internal, caused by a fractional increase in the salt content of the blood, upsetting the normal ratio of water and salt. A meal of salty ham or fish similarly can drive a person almost wild with thirst until the kidneys discharge the salt and get the blood ratio back into its proper range. These urges vanish, however, if the back of the throat is painted with an anesthetic solution.

Recent exploration of the brain with electrical probes has shown that the true site of the thirst sensation is a small region, the hypothalamus, close to the pituitary gland. Here we have strange little sense organs that monitor the water-to-salt ratio in the blood coursing through capillary beds of the carotid artery. A decrease in this proportion measuring no more than one to two per cent below normal apparently starts messages along an indirect route. From the hypothalamus the response may be an unidentified hormone to which the lining cells in the back of the throat are sensitive. Once stimulated by it, however, the throat cells relay nerve messages to the cerebral cortex and induce the conscious senses of thirst. No wonder we are vague about this "feeling." In reaching a better understanding of it, the scientists have also been able to contradict the old adage about leading a horse to water. Now they *can* make it drink, by sending electrical stimuli along fine wires to its hypothalamus. The animal will become so thirsty, in fact, as to return compulsively to the watering trough even right after it has drunk its unstimulated fill!

Satisfying thirst is a matter of getting the water-to-salt ratio in the blood back into the proper range. This can be accomplished by eating juicy fruits just as successfully as by drinking water or other liquids. In tropical countries where the water supplies are often contaminated, our own preference is to rely upon oranges and other fruits we can peel rather than boil water from public supplies for twenty minutes or treat it with chemicals. This method can prevent the development of thirst even where the air is so dry that seven to nine quarts of water are lost into it daily by evaporation from skin and lungs.

All of us are limited in the number of ways we can maintain the water-to-salt ratio in the blood by the comparative inefficiency of human kidneys and by our lack of special salt-secreting glands. We cannot manage as a seal does on a diet of raw fishes, chiefly because our kidneys require in flushing out products of protein digestion more water than can be gained from the fish flesh. A seal, by contrast, is efficient in excreting nitrogenous wastes, and the animal conserves water by losing none in the form of sweat. Nor can we drink sea water, as albatrosses and many bony fishes do, because we would have to excrete more water than we take in merely to get rid of the added salt. Each quart of sea water contains about thirty-five grams of salt; to get rid of it we would have to discharge nearly two quarts of liquid. The albatross and other tube-nosed birds drink sea water with impunity because their nostrils contain special glands which extract from the blood all superfluous salts and let them drip away in mucus to the outside world. Bony fishes in the sea achieve the same end with salt-secreting cells in the surface of the gills.

No mammals are known to make a habit of drinking sea water as a source of moisture. Yet the desert-dwelling kangaroo rats can be trained to do so. They are adapted in many peculiar ways to living where free water of any kind is rarely encountered. Kangaroo rats avoid the dry air of day, and even keep themselves from losing water by carrying any air-dried seeds to their burrows in fur-lined cheek pouches. In the burrow the trophies absorb water vapor from the soil, and the kangaroo rat then eats them. It is efficient in conserving water by re-absorbing the precious material in its kidneys until its liquid waste is more than twice as salty as sea water. Metabolic water can then suffice, letting the animal live its whole life without a drink. To a kangaroo rat, a sip of sea water represents surplus water, whereas to us it is merely extra salt.

Probably the camel could manage on sea water almost as well as the kangaroo rat. A camel's adaptations are many, and make us wonder why man's body could not be fitted similarly to conserving precious water. Yet most of its specializations are beyond human reach. We cannot let our bodies chill down to 95 degrees Fahrenheit in the cool desert night, to warm up slowly in the morning sun and reach a temperature of 105 degrees before we begin to sweat. We cannot route from the liver to the stomach (rather than the kidneys) a large part of our nitrogenous wastes, and reuse the material in synthesis of proteins—as the camel seems to do. If we could, it would save us from throwing away valuable water, and at the same time reduce the incidence of protein deficiency (kwashiorkor)—one of the world's most widespread diseases today. We cannot even conserve the water in our blood stream while losing it from the rest of the body's reserve, as a camel does. After seventeen days without water, a camel is very much alive, although it may have lost a tenth of its plasma water and a third of its other body water; it can recoup its losses in ten minutes if given access to a drinking trough.

Almost the only way in which we can imitate the camel is by wearing layer after layer of loose wool garments in the desert sun as the Arabs do, shielding the skin from the heat and reducing the need for water loss by perspiration to cool the skin. The camel's thick hair, sticking out several inches over surfaces exposed to the sun, is only part of this adaptation, however. The remainder lies in the camel's distribution of fat, which is largely restricted to the hump on its back rather than spread uniformly below the skin where we store so much. By the time a camel's body temperature has risen to 105 degrees, its skin surface is at about 103 and the outward flow of heat is relatively unimpeded. We can achieve equal dissipation of heat only by cooling the body surface five degrees or more through evaporation of sweat, costing us water we may have difficulty replacing. Yet without this cooling, the fatty insulation below the skin's surface so limits heat flow that our body temperature would rise to dangerous levels.

Seemingly the camel's adaptations include also a superior ability to identify acceptable water. It will readily take bitter solutions we would refuse except as a last resort. In deciding whether water is fit to drink, we rely heavily upon odor and taste, particularly upon the receptors affected by salt. Yet these too can fool us. Curiously, we show a preference for solutions containing traces of salt. Pure water, which we describe as "tasteless and odorless," we may even shun as "flat" and "uninteresting" in flavor.

At the Veterinary College in Stockholm, Dr. Yngve Zotterman and his colleagues have discovered that the frog's tongue possesses special taste endings that respond specifically to water and to highly dilute solutions of sodium chloride. Does this mean that the frog detects water as a distinct taste? The Swedish scientists suggest that the frog has this ability, and uses it in detecting any leakage of fresh water into the mouth when immersed. Since frogs do hide themselves in the muddy bottoms of ponds during winter months, the idea seems reasonable. But does man detect a specific taste in water, other than through identification of salt, sweet, sour, bitter or odorous materials dissolved in it?

No one seems to know what gave a tin dipperful of farm spring water its delicious taste. It wasn't the dipper alone, for the same utensil used to raise a sample of distilled water to the lips fails to conceal the striking difference. Most people who perform this test are ready to agree that really pure water is fine for automobile batteries, but scarcely fit to drink. Rain water, which is sun-distilled, shows the same lack of character. Even spring water that has stood for weeks in a closed glass container has a "livelier" flavor.

It is strange that we should react in this way for, more

than anything else, fresh water supplies determine where man can live. We recognize today not only personal thirst, but also civic thirst and industrial thirst. The growth of a city is determined by the extent to which its water supply can be augmented. The success of many industries, from steel-making to farming, depends upon the availability of vast amounts of water.

In the United States today, each man, woman and child shares in a demand averaging 200 gallons of fresh water per person per year for drinking, 15,000 gallons per person per year for washing, cooking and operating our living quarters, plus 160,000 gallons per person per year for industrial purposes, and 230,000 gallons per person per year for irrigation. For 180 million people, this amounts to about a seventh of all the water that runs down our streams and rivers into the ocean. With a predicted population of 360 million in the year 2000, a comparable thirst at private, civic and industrial levels will total a third of the fresh waters available.

Before too many years pass, man must either devise salt-extracting machines to let him produce fresh water from sea water, or find human populations along our coasts curbed by chronic thirst. Even then, the transport of large amounts of desalted sea water to the dry interiors of great continents is unlikely to be worth while economically—not on the scale required by agriculture, industry and large cities. Inland communities seemingly must depend indefinitely upon satisfying thirst from natural rainfall. In the future they may become fresh-water oases, with man hurrying from one to the next—perhaps wishing he were as well equipped to do so as a camel.

IV

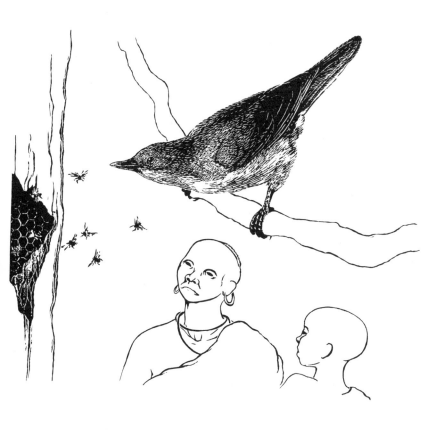

13. *Obscure Senses*

A GREAT change is needed in our attitude toward the human brain because of recent discoveries. No longer can we consider this center of consciousness and unwitting control for the body as merely an intricate telephone switchboard between senses and muscles or glands. It is not enough to grant that the brain serves also as a computer, and as a magnetic tape recorder with a lifetime supply of tape, giving us memory. It is true that we can still argue about what is meant by the "mind," and are unwilling to spend time hunting for an anatomical site for the soul. But we have become convinced that our mental machinery conceals some obscure senses for which no special organs have yet been found.

157

Perhaps all of these misunderstood senses will prove to operate through a "pleasure center" located recently in the brain, found by exploring the deeper portions with electrical probes. Direct stimulation of the pleasure center seems to substitute for food and sex and companionship, to the point where the scientists who discovered the center fear the consequences for mankind if unscrupulous people should find a way to market a self-stimulator reaching this region of the brain.

These discoveries seem a long way from the Sermon on the Mount and the beatitude "Blessed are they which do hunger and thirst after righteousness." Yet we must admit the reality of compelling inner forces, whether we call them cravings, desires, hungers, longings, passions or appetites. Our realization of a need for food, however vague it is, fits this description. So do our hidden urges to achieve security, to find companions or a mate, and to dream.

A few years ago, speculations on these characteristics of the human mind would have been regarded as idle and unscientific. Now they are open fields for serious inquiry. We can pursue them much farther than we used to. Using a whole array of instruments (including electroencephalographs to record "brain waves"), scientists have found that dreaming is an essential part of sleep if it is to knit "up the ravell'd sleave of care." Space physiologists find that the human brain must have a variety of stimulation while awake, and are concerned today with providing activities and entertainment for confined astronauts in interstellar space. Psychologists, moreover, have realized just recently that we require a quota of social bumps and bruises, acquired through parental handling and contacts with companions, if we are to develop a well-adjusted attitude to the world around us. Now when someone remarks that we should find satisfaction in the fact that the nervous system supervises so many different internal activities without distracting us from senses attuned to the outside world, we can both agree and also ask: "Is satisfaction a sense too?" It may be akin to a "sense" of beauty or a feeling of affection. How many vague senses of this type can we find concealed just below our consciousness?

FOOD

How vague is a sense of needing food? As mealtime
approaches, we involuntarily grow restless, shift our feet,
squirm in our chairs, and show a reduced ability to concentrate on work. Our stomach may begin fairly rhythmic
contractions that increase in vigor and frequency until we
detect them as "hunger pangs." The distinguished physiologists W. B. Cannon and A. L. Washburn, who began
measuring these contractions, claimed in 1912 that hunger
was merely a conscious consequence of the "pangs." Their
claim has since been disproved, for people whose stomachs
have been removed surgically still feel hunger (although
not hunger pangs), and all of us continue to want more
food after the first few mouthfuls have progressed to the
stomach and stilled its signaling. We can agree with the
seventeenth-century Archbishop Fénelon of Cambrai, that
"cookery is the art of... rendering the appetite still im-
portunate, when the wants of nature are supplied."

No one has identified the basis for appetite. It is not
simply a vague awareness that the concentration of sugar
in the blood has fallen. Nor can a "hunger hormone" be
ruled out yet as a partial explanation, for a transfusion of
blood from a hungry dog into a well-fed one will make the
satiated animal eager for food again. Blood from a well-fed
dog similarly will quiet the hunger pangs in a hungry
animal—for a few minutes.

Any adequate explanation of appetite must account
both for its impelling character and also its often-specific
direction. We recall one craving that developed while we
were patrons at an English guesthouse in Jamaica, B.W.I.
From immediately after breakfast until just before dinner
at night, we were out on field work each day, usually with
a big carton of sandwiches and fresh fruit. The breakfast
was hearty, with hot or cold cereal, eggs, potatoes, toast
and tea. The meat or cheese sandwiches and the lunch
fruit were delicious. The dinner seemed all we could ask
for—except for dessert. The trifles and puddings and occasional tipsy cakes were all just barely sweet. We continued
automatically in our habit of adding no sugar to anything

at the table—none on fruit or cereal or in a beverage.

Within two weeks we became aware of an intense yearning for jam, candy, ice cream or other food sweeter than Jell-O. We knew we were eating big meals, and yet the longing grew almost unbearable. A pound of English toffee did not relieve it. Then came some rainy weather that confined us in the afternoons and introduced us to teatime. We're afraid we weren't well mannered, for we ignored the carefully buttered squares of thin-sliced, crust-free bread. We wolfed the sweet cakes that were supposed to follow, reveling in the icing—and salvaging every crumb of it. Suddenly we realized that this sugar hunger never develops in our own home, because of the frequency with which we enjoy sweet coffee cake or jam-on-toast for breakfast, or indulge in a really sweet dessert at lunch or dinner. We wonder now whether comparable cravings would develop in an environment affording us a curtailment in fats or almost no proteins. How discriminating can hungers be?

Friends have told us that, while awake and also in their dreams at night, they longed for a glass of cold milk after only a few weeks where none could be had. Seemingly no sense reminded them of the drink they missed. And yet we wonder how different this pointed hunger is from the seductive appeal an ex-smoker feels for years, whenever his nose picks up the spicy scent of a freshly opened package of cigarettes. The odor of tobacco smoke itself may come to repel him, without altering the insistent lure of that once-familiar fragrance.

We wonder too what sensory system or nervous center leads a female mosquito (but not her mate) to seek a blood meal from specific kinds of warm-blooded animals. Certainly it is a protein hunger, for she searches out a victim whose blood proteins she can digest. From the products she produces nitrogen-rich compounds needed for normal development of her eggs.

The mosquito's travels, which may take her on tortuous routes over an area two miles across, are powered mainly with energy from sugar in nectar she drinks from flowers along the way. Yet, as she stops for a sip, she remains alert for a warm-bodied neighbor. Her choice of a victim includes a good many kinds from among the birds and mammals of the region. A mosquito that would feed on lemmings in a year of their abundance has to be able to accept blood from a reindeer or a sleeping bird when lemmings are scarce.

Formerly it was believed that failure to locate a suitable source of blood left a mosquito barren. Recently, however, mosquitoes were found able to produce small batches of eggs without a blood meal, by mobilizing protein resources from within the insect's own body. These come from small bits of larval tissues remaining between the adult organs. Some kinds of Scandinavian mosquitoes, at least, can also digest their own flight muscles in the thorax after prolonged searching has failed to satisfy the hunger for fresh blood.

If we cannot reach a satisfying explanation for the hungers we all feel from time to time, how can we expect to account for the more esoteric hungers we observe in other creatures? Particularly puzzling are those animals that devour quantities of materials for which they themselves have no digestive agents. How did certain cockroaches and termites evolve the custom of devouring dry wood and paper, or one little group of robin-sized birds an analogous taste for beeswax in the forests from South Africa to Borneo?

Both these particular insects and the unusual birds, to be sure, have intestinal microbes able to utilize the indigestible substances, able to convert cellulose into starches and sugars or wax into digestible residues. Yet the problem remains. Which came first: the intestinal partners or the choice of indigestible foodstuffs? Did the wood roaches and the wood-eating termites become social in their habits as a means for conveying an internal legacy of cellulose-splitting microbes from one generation to the next? Or did insects for which social organization had other significance acquire intestinal microbes that permitted a change of diet to one of pure cellulose?

The wood roaches and termites are completely consistent about their strange diet, for they take to it immediately after hatching from the egg. The wax-eating birds of the Old World, by contrast, have no opportunity to indulge their bizarre taste until almost fully grown. Each of them is a foundling foisted upon foster parents, much in the manner of the European cuckoo. Once abroad on its own, however, the wax-hungry bird begins to visit bees' nests that have been ripped apart by badgerlike ratels, or by native people. Soon a new phase of this habit appears: the bird becomes a winged pilot, chirping and attracting the attention of ratels and natives. For as much as thirty-minute expeditions, it will lead them to a bee tree. From this the birds gain their English name "honeyguides" and their scientific category—the genus *Indicator*. Recently the key to the story fell into place for these birds. Honeyguides acquire the bacterial partner, together with a yeast, from wild honeycomb. An unknown cofactor, furnished by the bird's digestive tract, allows the bacteria and the yeast to work together on beeswax, breaking it down rapidly into relatively simple fatty acids useful to the bird as well as nutrients important to the microbes. The partnership arises freshly in each almost-grown honeyguide. But the bird's obvious hunger for wax remains a riddle.

Despite the fact that huge molecules, such as those of wax and cellulose, are virtually insoluble in water or saliva, there is always the possibility that they have a flavor or odor which an animal can detect. Birds are less likely than cockroaches to be able to rely upon smell or taste, for few birds have more than a token representation of the needed sense organs. Still, the critical sensitivities might be present.

Neither taste nor smell, however, explains a hunger. What tells a bird that the pebbles embedded in the walls of its gizzard have worn smooth and small? For a bird to swallow pieces of rock deliberately may be reasonable to us when we know that the grinding action of the gizzard depends upon the presence of these hard particles. But what triggers the instinctive act of eating pebbles? How did such an instinct develop? What of the giant dinosaurs of the Age of Reptiles, which armed their gizzards with rock fragments as big as a man's clenched fist? Fossil hunters find these "gastroliths" today, and know how they were worn smooth. Even though a dinosaur might be able to find a flavor difference between a chunk of limestone and a block of granite, its urge to swallow either remains astonishing.

So many actions of animals serve a purpose that the

origins of instinctive actions become tantalizing topics. Scientists are convinced that nonhuman life does not first identify a need and then go about satisfying it. We prefer, instead, to believe that the actions we see represent learning from fortuitous experiences of the individual, or that they arose as inborn features through random mutations which proved to be valuable adaptations.

Rather often we remain uncertain which explanation accounts for an animal's behavior. Is it "play" or "practice" or something still obscure that keeps a well-fed cat eager for the chase, capturing and killing mice or small birds? In the wild, a honeyguide similarly will often lead the way to a bee tree and then perch near by without adding a morsel to the cropful of beeswax remaining from an earlier meal. The bird may even fly away before its appetite returns. Any realistic explanation of appetite must account for these animals that, when satiated, still continue with actions providing more food. Probably the correct interpretation of the facts will be the key also to the actions of the man who, after making a fortune, continues working as hard as when he was poor. Surely it can't be habit alone!

SEX

Food takes on a very different importance in the various animals, from insects to man, in which the male offers something edible as a gift to the potential mate he is pursuing. This link between taste, olfactory sense and sex is conspicuous when a man brings a box of candy to the woman of his choice. For the human species we often conclude that the gift shows that he would be a good provider, that he is ready to assume the responsibilities of supporting a family. Such a conclusion appears to suit modern examples in which parental care extends beyond its former limits. The American father who furnishes his son with a sports car during the dating years may differ only in degree from the man in Africa south of the Sahara who uses cattle as a medium of exchange for women— three heifers and two bulls for a bride for his son, or a similar bride price (*lobola*) for another wife for himself.

Perhaps this interpretation is biased and overlooks the original meaning in the custom. Among animals in which the male offers a free meal to a member of the opposite sex, it often serves merely to distract her and keep her quiet while he mates with her. At one extreme is the praying mantis, with the male himself becoming the gift of food for his cannibalistic mate. At the other may be the black-tipped hangingfly *Bittacus*, which feeds on mosquitoes, other small insects and spiders. The male *Bittacus* captures a fine juicy mosquito, presents it to a female, mates with her quickly while she feeds on it, then takes the remains of the prey away from her and offers them to other willing females in turn until the mosquito's internal juices have been drained and his "gift" loses its appeal.

The eminent entomologist William Morton Wheeler traced a whole series of gift-giving among various little flies. Some of them present a potential mate with an attractive bit of food. Others first carefully wrap the gift in a swaddling of silken secretion. Still others merely provide an empty package of silken strands, as a sort of toy balloon which distracts the female and buys her cooperation. In male flies that cautiously retrieve the toy after his mate tires of it and then use it to gain favors from another female, Wheeler saw a parallel to the human suitor who frugally takes back his engagement ring and fits it on another lady's finger.

Courtship antics of the male should lead to his satisfaction in possessing a mate. We can see the gain to the species from his persistence. In many instances, we know that he behaves as he does because he is stimulated by specific hormones circulating in his blood. But where in the nervous system are the sensory areas responding to this stimulus, orienting his activities toward the opposite sex? Until they are found, sexual appetite will remain an obscure sense even though it is so widespread in the animal kingdom.

Almost certainly the sense organs vital to sex are hidden deep in the nervous system. Presumably they develop or become useful when new linkages of nerve cells mature. In this way the timing of the male's awareness of sex matches achievement of his physical maturity. For most animals the maturing nervous system adds also a fresh array of instincts, which lead to correct and almost automatic use of the sex organs. Only mankind may need instruction and a few of his most thoroughbred domestic animals need actual help in mating. For the rest of the animal kingdom, the sexual instincts form an efficient chain of reactions, based on an inner urge as real as hunger or thirst or fear, and often stronger than any of these. Each step in the series can be expected to lead to a definite result, and that result to form the stimulus for the next step. If any step is blocked, the rest of the chain may go unused until a way around the obstacle is found.

Often other senses set the instinctive chain in motion. The odor or sight or sound of a female starts the male in a direction which, with her co-operation, leads to fertilization of her sex cells. Only that final event is important. But devious indeed are the sensory complications in getting a sperm to an egg for the final conquest!

Sex is important because the versatile, rather than the meek, inherit the earth. Our own chances of survival are enhanced if mankind includes a large number of different types rather than only one. Each male, by his contribution, adds immeasurably to variation among his offspring. In this way he insures the versatility that will be tested by the environment as we battle the present for the right to a future.

Among our fellow creatures, the male may be small. His life may be brief. But the effects of his sexual appetite are enormous. Usually it makes him ready, able and willing to mate with almost any co-operative female. She, by contrast, has the onerous task of producing eggs, and often of caring for the young. His timing must be suited to hers. Often courtship serves, through her responses, to advise the male when she is ready to accept him. To these responses, all his senses may be alerted.

Even when the female's physical condition is right she may not be aware of it. In animals whose behavior is a network of instincts, the whole of life may be compartmented into actions based upon the internal stimulus of hunger, or the external stimulus of food or of fear, or the partly internal, partly external stimulus of sex. Courtship by the male helps the female make the transition from one of these compartmented awarenesses to that of sex. Once this has been accomplished, in fact, she may be sufficiently aroused to be eager to mate with any male that comes along.

Partly because most of the scientists investigating sexual behavior have been men, from Freud to Kinsey, the female remains in many instances a baffling enigma. So often her actions, which excite the male, appear to be trivial demonstrations of her femininity engaged in only for her own entertainment. Nobel laureate Anatole France made this clear in his delightful allegory *Penguin Island*, particularly when the Devil (in the guise of a respected monk) draped clothes for the first time on a young female penguin. Despite the ceaseless accumulation of male penguins panting after her, "she went on peacefully and seemed to see nothing."

Whether or not human civilization arose as Anatole France described satirically, courtship among primitive peoples often follows a pattern almost as fixed as the instinctive behavior of nonhuman animals. Seemingly, for all his inventiveness, man has hit upon few techniques for gaining a lady's favor that have not been used in infinite variety by the smaller creatures he so frequently overlooks. Yet one difference stands out. Except in the human species, females are ordinarily masters of the situation: the male cannot mate with them unless they co-operate. The solitary human female, however, is peculiarly vulnerable to attack by males whose sexual interests have been aroused. This difference probably ranks beside our greatly extended childhood as a reason for the development of prolonged parental care, of co-operating family groups and of civilization itself.

SECURITY

The response of a female to sex hunger is channeled along very different routes from that of a male, and usually is linked to another obscure sense—the sense of security. We can call it assurance, or self-confidence, or faith, or even by the old word "spirit." It still relates in both sexes to an awareness of self in relation to the world that is just as real (although deeply hidden) as the mental picture of our environment that we build with information from eyes, ears, and organs of touch. An underdeveloped sense of security is the torment of the chronically timid and fearful.

For the female, this sense is bound up closely with her role as a provider for the young, particularly in kinds of animals that build a nest or protect the offspring in some way. New ways to measure these differences between the sexes continue to turn up. For mankind, a special feature has been found recently concealed somewhere in the computer mechanism of the brain's visual centers. This department is linked to the nervous pathways controlling the size of the pupil—the opening in the iris through which light enters the important back chamber of the eye. In response to the brain's identification of objects with special personal interest, the pupils increase as much as 17 per cent in diameter. For a woman, a picture of a mother and baby has greatest appeal—more than the baby alone. Men give almost no response to photographs of babies or of mothers with infants, but show a strong interest in landscape pictures—subjects toward which most women give a negative reaction. As might be expected, photographs of nude members of the opposite sex cause a prompt widening of the pupils, whereas those of members of the same sex lack interest.

How early these sexual differences in interest appear is still unknown. But at the University of Wisconsin, Dr. Harry F. Harlow has been measuring the beginnings of the sense of security in infant monkeys as they soak up self-confidence from their surrogate "mothers" merely through contact with the terry-cloth covering and the act of clinging with arms reached around "her." The speed with which the baby can become reassured when an unfamiliar object is thrust into the test cage seems increased if the "mother" rocks back and forth gently. How many external senses serve as avenues to the same hidden center in the brain, building courage "to the sticking place"?

A baby chick stimulates its own sense of security by

hiding under the mother hen. A baby rhinoceros runs from danger to the farther side of its bulky mother. Our own self-confidence is noticeably greater in the security of our homes. We might conclude that the ancestors of today's Englishmen set out so bravely to conquer the world because their homes had been made legally as secure as castles. The inviolate home became a sort of surrogate mother. In many countries, this source of security is safeguarded into modern times by adopted English laws.

Companionship is important too in the proper functioning of the sense of security. The little monkeys that developed "baby love" for a cloth-covered stick in Wisconsin failed to mature into normal adults. Without the care they would have received—and cuffs from a mother whose patience they had exhausted—they never learned to groom themselves or even to show real interest in other monkeys. In the jungle, monkeys are in frequent playful contact with one another. They compensate for the lack of a home by seeking safety in numbers.

An astonishing number of unlike animals find companionship important. Many butterflies and bats seek out sleeping places close to others of their own kind. Migrating grasshoppers and birds commonly travel in groups. Bumblebees and purple martins nest where they have near neighbors. Antelopes and rabbits usually feed companionably in the dark. The outcast from a herd, in fact, often becomes a rogue and deteriorates physically as though ready to die from loneliness.

In a homeless outcast, the psychiatrist might recognize the symptoms of an inferiority complex, with evidences of insecurity increasing in proportion to the extent of trespass on the territory of integrated herds. Alternatively, the blundering destruction or timid hesitation might be compared to the movements of a person in complete darkness or on unfamiliar ground. Perhaps the pathways serving the sense of security in the outcast's brain are no longer bringing the needed stimuli, and the actions of the lonely one are a logical outcome.

A variety of chemical substances can reach the obscure centers of our sense of security. Tranquilizers seem to operate in this way. Nor are these therapeutic materials designed to relieve human tensions without precedent in the animal kingdom. A unifying tranquilizer, secreted by the queen honeybee, is responsible for maintaining the whole organization of a beehive. The workers cannot manage without it. Today we know the chemical constitution of the compound, but not why the workers like it, or how they distribute it so democratically, or in what ways it focuses each bee's attention on instinctive drives in proper sequence—as though the nervous system issued a new day's instructions every morning.

We wonder, too, where in the bee's tiny brain "queen substance" has its effect. Surely these cells will prove to be a counterpart of our hypothalamus—the center in which most of our obscure senses lie concealed, close to the connection with our pituitary gland. For our hypothalamus to possess these sensory roles seems logical, since it is derived from the same part of the brain in the developing embryo as the light-sensitive part of the eyes. Evolution has carried the retinas outward to an association with a cornea and lens derived from the skin, and hence to a role related directly to the outside world. The remaining sensory functions of this region in the human brain have developed in association with other parts of the body. They can be thought of as "looking" inward. To this they owe their complex role in the mature individual.

As usual, science has answered vague questions by raising a wonderful array of better questions. They penetrate farther, and also reveal more orderliness and "rightness" in the universe. No one aspect of science has such appeal for the scientist as this orderliness and rightness. Each new discovery that fits neatly into place in an old theory appeals directly to the sense of security. So does the underlying simplicity of natural laws. Both produce a glow of intellectual satisfaction that is international, independent of time and place, and contagious.

SLEEP AND DREAMS

The human brain conceals in the hypothalamus still other obscure senses for which no special centers have been found. One of them reaches away from reality and the confines of circumstances, and seems most active during sleep. Sleep too is centered in the hypothalamus. But what is sleep? Is it a basic resting condition, from which we can be roused for limited lengths of time by varied stimulation? None of the several theories that have been offered gives a satisfactory account of this regularly recurring period of unconsciousness. None of them explains why even voluntary wakefulness leads, after between thirty and sixty hours, to profound psychological changes such as loss of memory, hallucinations, and even fragmentation of the personality. None of them shows why healthy adult cattle and sheep appear able to manage with little or no sleep—although certain advantages can be seen in connection with the complicated digestive processes of cud-chewing animals.

To be adequate, any theory of sleep must show what this condition means to a butterfly or a bee, to a snail or an octopus, as well as to a fish or a crocodile. These, like birds and most mammals, require for health a number of hours in each twenty-four spent in inactivity—even if they have no eyelids to close. They need it in the tropics, where day and night are approximately equal, and near the poles, where first day and then night reaches a length of twenty-four hours.

What obscure sense do we try to ignore after a good meal, when we resist the urge to sleep as so many animals do, letting the increased stomach activity during this type of unconsciousness improve our digestion? What kind of monitoring inner eye scans our sensory horizons to learn whether all is quiet? For mankind the ideal conditions for sleep are a darkened room, a familiar bed, still air and silence—or a soft lullaby—all benefits our remote ancestors could have found in caves.

Perhaps we are putting the emphasis in the wrong place. The magic of sleep may lie neither in improved digestion nor in obvious unconsciousness, but in an opportunity to dream freely. Can we take a fresh look at Hamlet's fears: "To sleep! perchance to dream"? Psychologists at the University of Chicago are now wondering if dreams may be as necessary as sleep. With Dr. Nathaniel Kleitman and other experimenters as subjects, they are attaching electrical connections to the scalp and face near the eyes, then recording the activities of brain and closed eyes by means of electronic devices. By awakening the sleeper as soon as the record pattern shows that dreaming has begun, they can reduce total dreaming time by 75 to 80 per cent. After a few days of this treatment, emotional composure declines. Anxiety, increased irritability and other symptoms usually associated with sleeplessness appear. No comparable changes follow if sleepers are awakened with equal frequency, but between dreams. Dr. Charles Fisher at Mount Sinai Hospital in New York City is reported to have suggested that "dreaming permits each and every one of us to be quietly and safely insane every night of our lives."

Some people claim that they never dream. Others remember their fantasies vividly, or even rouse themselves when the unconscious mind imagines situations that are too exciting or too unbelievable. Seemingly the sleeping brain plays games. It matches together fragments of memory and interprets the unlikely combinations in ways we would inhibit while awake. Apparently every human being dreams. The "nonrecallers" realize this with surprise when they are awakened repeatedly in mid-dream—a state recognizable both from the tracings of their brain waves and from jerky scanning movements of their closed eyes. These objective signs of dreaming were discovered first in studies on the sleep of infants. Mere babies reach a stage in sleep like that of adults, at which major body movements cease and the closed eyes commence to rove as though following objects of interest. When the dream ends, the eyes become quiet, and body movements usually reappear.

Adults may erase all recollection of a dream by having afterward ten minutes of uninterrupted sleep. Rarely do dreams lead to any muscular action. The messages that would cause us to do something while awake seem to fade out on their way from the sleeping brain to the muscles. Sleepwalkers appear to be exceptional. To this extent their brain is acting as though it were awake. For other people, the mind must be conscious to compare experiences and generate a response in the form of action—or lack of action, by "not doing what comes naturally"!

But what of sleep in other animals? Must they also dream? A dog, sleeping in front of the fire, often lies on his side with eyes closed and ears limp, yet twitches his feet and engages in little sniffing movements, as though enjoy ing a hunting fantasy in his sleep. Caged birds, without appearing to awaken, sometimes sing softly day or night, with eyes tightly closed. Are they too dreaming?

Solving these riddles seems likely to uncover a host of other obscure senses, and to show still more features that all life holds in common. Almost certainly, however, some answers will come intuitively, during dreams. The German chemist Friedrich August Kekule von Stradonitz, who, had he lived another decade, might have been awarded a Nobel prize for proposing the ring form of the benzene molecule, told how this radical idea came to him in a dream. In his fantasy, imagined molecules were dancing about, some of them with the shape of snakes. One of these whirling snake molecules seized its own tail in its mouth. "Like a flash of lightning," Kekule's sleeping mind recognized that here lay the explanation for the puzzling properties of benzene! "Learn to dream, gentlemen," he wrote later. "Then we shall, perhaps, find the truth. We must take care, however, not to publish our dreams before submitting them to proof by the awakened mind."

How many of us have dreamed, in sleep or while half-awake, that our bodies somehow took wings and soared through the air? A ride in a jet airplane does not satisfy this wish, even though the airplane itself seems the tangible, working outcome of science fiction. Fiction of all kinds has the form of published dreams, some of which are recognized as prophecy when they come true. We may ask how far civilization would have come toward modern times without skilled dreamers in the past. In ways we still do not understand, they put to use an obscure sensory area of the brain, finding a way into a different future—one no outward sense could yet detect.

When we dream, we free our minds from the limitations of the present reality and enter an imaginary world that is like, but not identical with, the one we know. In the differences between this dream world and the real one (where everything is unique—like nothing else), we glimpse a part of our own personality that is hidden deeper than any of the obscure senses in the hypothalamus. It is our subconscious self, whose effects upon our conscious actions are too subtle to be noticed except on rare occasions.

Sleep lets our subconscious self be active. But can we call it forth even momentarily while awake? Sometimes, when we have puzzled long over a difficult decision and see no clear action on the basis of our information, we toss a coin. Immediately chance has indicated the choice, we know from our own elation or disappointment what our subconscious prefers. If only we could understand the relationship between our obscure senses and our subconscious in the decisions we make, many of the riddles in our lives would promptly solve themselves.

V

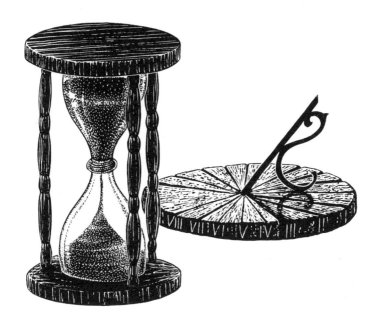

14. *What Time Is It?*

How OFTEN, after setting the alarm clock to awaken us at some unusual hour, we suddenly regain consciousness from a relaxing sleep just a minute or less before the signal rings out! The clock gives us no prior warning click, and we are relying upon its bell as on a faithful servant. Many people need not even set a clock. At a self-appointed hour they awaken as though in response to an inner clockwork.

Perhaps a majority of us accomplish the same end because we arise regularly at some definite time of day. Often we shrug this off as habit, forgetting that the brain does not act as a self-timer—telling us merely when we have had some constant number of sleeping hours. Our inner clock is far more remarkable than any hour glass. It follows the twenty-four-hour cycle and remains reasonably independent of the hour of retiring. If we set it unconsciously for six-thirty every morning, it nudges us into awakening close to that hour unless we have let ourselves become utterly fatigued late the night before.

It is entirely possible that, by inventing mechanical clocks and relying upon them, we have largely forgotten how to use a living clock mechanism inside our nervous system. Dr. Gustav Eckstein tells a charming story about the late Swiss composer Emile Jaques-Dalcroze, who used to entertain his son and self while walking together in the evenings. The father held his watch in his hand. He waited until it showed that a new minute was about to begin. Then suddenly he covered the watch face and said "three" (or some other number of his choice, as the time interval to be estimated). After a period of silence as they walked, father and son would call "three"—usually simultaneously. And the father would uncover the watch face and see how close their estimates had been. Jaques-Dalcroze insisted that anyone could do as well at this game, if only they would relax and ignore the outer clock.

One Christmas season we were quartered in the Pan-American Agricultural School at Zamorano, Republic of Honduras. Most of the Spanish-speaking students were still present, for the simple reason that the scholarships on which they had come from distant areas did not pay their way home for the holidays. And so the campus was lively, each evening given over to group discussions in some dormitory rooms and impromptu musicals in others. Groups of boys gathered wherever three or four or five of them had marimbas. At first, each player would warm up with a solo number, a melodious rhythm of his own choosing. Then some selection would catch the fancy of the others, and suddenly as though a great orchestra had been switched on, the trio or quartet or quintet would burst into action. As a team they hammered away, playing parts and intricate variations, all with no pages of music and no conductor to keep the exhilarating tempo. Six hands, eight hands, ten hands, each striking at the proper instant or poised, waiting through those syncopated pauses so characteristic of Latin music, before snapping down again at the exact split second.

For the human body to possess an inner metronome of this kind is less surprising than if we lacked one. Virtually every kind of animal has a timing system, as a personal chronometer against which to regulate its life. Many of these living clocks run with remarkable accuracy for days or weeks after the animals containing them are placed in laboratory surroundings made unvarying in every way anyone can think of. Light intensity can be constant. So can sound level, humidity, barometric pressure, and the availability of the same assortment of foods. Temperature is less critical, for the living clocks are almost all well compensated against slow temperature changes within the range from near freezing to slightly above the warmth of human blood.

All of the clock mechanisms in living things must have a chemical form. Certainly a complex nervous system is not required, for plants and single-celled organisms show time-keeping abilities too. So far, however, animals have been examined in far greater detail in a determined hunt to find the elusive internal chronometer.

The little fruit fly *Drosophila*, which passes so easily through the fine mesh of window screens and hovers around ripe fruit in the house, ordinarily reaches adulthood about an hour before dawn. It will do so even if kept in continual darkness after the initial day of its three-to-four-day maggothood, through the four-to-five-day pupal period during which the tissues of the yeast-eating maggot stage are converted over into the body of the winged adult. Emergence just before dawn lets the little fly take advantage of the highest relative humidity predictable for the day. The soft-bodied fly can expand to full diminutive size and harden its waterproof exterior before dry air steals away its minute store of moisture.

If fruit-fly eggs are placed in the dark and the flies allowed to develop there, the adults show none of this synchronized emergence from the pupa. To set its clock the maggot of the pupa must receive at least one brief flash of light, simulating dawn, more than two days before readiness to emerge to adulthood. Ordinarily the insect rechecks the setting of its timing mechanism day after day, in relation to dawn. But if necessary the fly will develop in the dark without changing from its original setting, until it has completed preparations for emergence; then it will wait until the internal clock signals the correct hour of the twenty-four for the final transformation.

Comparable internal clocks running on solar time are evident in the feeding habits of many animals. Cockroaches in a dark storeroom keep to a definite schedule. Mosquitoes in equatorial Africa bite according to a time scale often as restricted as thirty minutes in a twenty-four-hour day; it may come at the end of evening twilight, or at midnight, or in the early-morning hours, according to the particular kind of mosquito. Honeybee workers rest quietly in the darkness of the hive until the hours when their favorite flowers are freshly opening with a new supply of nectar; then out the insects go to gather the sweet juice. As the season progresses, they adjust their internal clocks to the particular plants blossoming.

Our own mealtimes are important to us in relation to a twenty-four-hour internal clock. If we travel by fast airplane either east or west, we reach places where noon comes earlier or later than we are used to. A traveler may have a quick breakfast in New York before boarding a westbound jet, be served a second breakfast aboard and, when he arrives on the West Coast, find people just sitting down to breakfast there—asking him to join them at an hour when his stomach calls for lunch. Hours for retiring and arising are displaced too from the habitual times he has been following. Usually the traveler needs several days to reset his internal clock to the new schedule. By slower means of transportation the adjustment could be made with less impact, for meals and sleeping time would come only an hour or two earlier or later each day and hence fit into the scale of ordinary variation in living habits.

Some comfort may be found in scientific proof that other animals with internal clocks are equally out-of-step with local time when they are transported rapidly east and west. A two-way shipment of bees was made by fast airplane to see whether the insects would reset their timing mechanisms in the darkened containers en route. But the Parisian bees stayed on Paris time in New York City, and the New York bees on New York time in Paris, until new stimuli showed them the need for an adjustment to match unfamiliar routines of feeding and sleeping.

Recently the site of the internal clock was discovered for one kind of insect: exactly four special cells embedded below the tiny brain of a cockroach. By careful surgery these cells can be removed and transplanted to another cockroach, without upsetting the timing mechanism. We might take as the donor an ordinary cockroach whose clock cells call for activity between 6 P.M. and 6 A.M., when the storeroom lights are out. Don Marquis' character Archie was just such an insect. The recipient of the transplant could be a laboratory cockroach whose clock has become adjusted to life in a place where lamps burn brightly—inhibiting activity—all night, but where the shades are drawn and food is available from 6 A.M. to 6 P.M. After the surgical work, the laboratory cockroach with the clock cells from the ordinary roach in place of its own would hide away all day and become active at 6 P.M., even in continuous darkness or under constant dim light.

Man's mechanical clocks and watches are regulated to divide the twenty-four-hour day accurately between successive times when the sun appears to cross the north-south vertical plane from pole to pole. If any more distant star is used instead of the sun as a reference point, the recurrent passage through the meridian comes 235.91 seconds early, as measured by sun-time clocks. Chronometers can be adjusted to match this slightly faster schedule and keep sidereal time. During the 365¼ solar days during which the earth circuits the sun, the succession of 235.91-second intervals add up to one whole solar day— one rotation of the earth unwound, so to speak, by the orbiting planet.

Astronomers find importance in sidereal time, for it helps them aim their telescopes accurately despite the movements of the orbiting earth. Only recently, however, were any animals found to have an internal clock keeping to a cycle 23 hours, 54 minutes, 4.09 seconds long as measured by our ordinary clocks and watches. Birds that migrate by night and use the stars for guidance apparently possess this internal rhythm and can employ it in navigating their way. This, and comparable use of cues from the sun's position, seem such astonishing awareness that they are regarded as part of a more complex direction sense.

For a very large number of different kinds of animals, as for man, a more immediate question in any coastal community is "When will the next high tide come?" We are well aware today that, under the influence of gravitational forces exerted by the moon and sun, ocean waters flow in patterns that produce tides. But as the moon circuits the earth, the earth rotates and orbits around the sun. The water movements are channeled by the continental contours and take time—introducing lags differing from place to place. At any given coastal point, one high tide follows another at approximately $12\frac{3}{4}$-hour intervals, with a low tide between them, more or less midway. It is far easier to draw up a set of tables than to construct a clock that will relate all of the variables and predict the tidal schedule a shellfisherman or an oyster needs to know.

An oyster has an internal clock that runs on tidal time. Shellfish dug from a New England bay and shipped in wet packing to a Midwest laboratory will continue to regulate their lives according to ocean tides nearly a thousand miles away. Gape of shell valves and consumption of oxygen increase and decrease in tempo with the flow and ebb of home waters, and not according to the schedule tides would follow if the Midwest were ocean-covered.

Fiddler crabs, on the other hand, obey both a solar and a tidal clock. They show the compounded rhythm in the hormone-controlled spread or contraction of pigment cells that dot the body surface. The fundamental solar rhythm, pale ivory-white by night and dark brownish gray by day, is accentuated by the tidal rhythm. The animal is still paler while the tide is high at night than when it is low, and still darker while the tide is low by day than when it is high. A fiddler crab hides in its burrow at high tide and emerges to feed at low. Supposedly it has better camouflage by being dark like the mud of the salt-marsh gutters where it scavenges for food during low tides in daylight.

When carried into the laboratory, fiddler crabs will continue their color changes in complete darkness or dim illumination, such as a full moon might give in their salt-marsh habitat. With practice anyone can learn to read the crab's clock by comparing its body color against a reference chart. From hourly records of pigment dispersal a graph can be drawn on which the interaction of the twenty-four-hour solar cycle and of the $12\frac{3}{4}$-hour tidal cycle becomes obvious.

Near Woods Hole Marine Biological Laboratory, where many studies of Massachusetts fiddler crabs have been made, these astonishing little animals can be collected either on the Buzzards Bay side or the Vineyard Sound shore of Cape Cod. The high tide reaches the gutters of the sound about four and a half hours before those of the bay. Fiddler crabs from these two localities, brought into the same faintly illuminated laboratory, continue each on its own compromise between solar and tidal cycles. They will do so even if shipped to the west coast of America or to Europe, unless at some time they are given a brief exposure to bright light—resetting their internal clocks for both rhythms simultaneously.

It is tempting for an investigator to look from a thick book of tide tables to a fiddler crab in a finger bowl and ask himself, "How can a little animal carry such a complex set of interlacing cycles in its body?" But the crab shows no real localization of its ability. Even an isolated leg, shed instinctively in the midst of a battle, will continue for a day or so to exhibit the color changes characteristic of the body as a whole—matching the solar and tidal rhythms without interruption. Only for the resetting of the internal clock must the crab have at least one eye and most of its nervous system intact. Thereafter the timekeeping seems to be transferred to tissues all over the body.

Familiar to beachcombers from Cape Hatteras into the West Indies and from San Pedro, California, to Panama are the wedge clams known as pompano shells or coquinas. They keep close account of tidal rhythms without adjusting their clocks on a solar rhythm too. On a rising tide, they respond to the acoustic shock of each breaking wave by kicking themselves out of the sand, letting the water carry them up the beach. As the wave recedes again, they quickly dig downward out of sight. On a falling tide, they emerge instead into the backwash of each wave, to be rolled down the beach again and complete the tide-triggered migration.

Fellow marine creatures, such as many sea worms and a few kinds of fishes, show a combined awareness of tidal rhythms, the phases of the moon, and the seasons. Their interacting internal clocks enable them to fit their mating

antics to a particular tide. Especially is this true of animals
that limit themselves to the night hours when the earth's
own shadow spreads safety upon the waters.

It is easy to understand how a palolo worm or a grunion
might avoid showing itself in daylight. More remarkable
but less obvious is the mechanism that allows it to match
its activities to both the 24.8-hour lunar day—measured
from moonrise to moonrise—and also the 29.5 day synodi-
cal month—measured from full moon to full moon. Yet in
the high tide at night in the third quarter of the moon in
October and again in November, the segmented palolo
worms of coral-reef crannies in the South Seas swarm at
the surface in such numbers that native people make these
dates a special feast night, with palolo worms as the
main dish.

We have watched a counterpart of the sea worms'
spawning along the California coast from Monterey
southward, just after the dark and the full of the moon.
The miracle is timed closely to match the hour of highest
spring tides at night. Only then do the smeltlike grunions
turn into acrobats, throwing themselves ashore—to the
delight of thousands of people who come to marvel, and
go home with buckets full of fish. Each female grunion
wiggles vertically downward tail first into the sand to lay
her eggs. At the same moment, one or two males curl about
her on the beach. Then out she squirms in time to travel
with her consorts back to the sea with the next wave. Not
for two weeks, unless there is a violent storm, will the surf
pound so high again on the land. And by then the grunion
eggs will have developed into young fish ready to explode
into the waves and join their parents in the Pacific. The
importance of this timing is evident. But how does a
grunion know what time it is?

In trying to discover what makes these living clocks tick,
scientists have progressed chiefly to finding out how to
stop or reset the mechanism. Anyone can temporarily halt
the timing system of an ant, merely by dropping the insect
into a light-proof box. The sudden and unusual change
quiets the ant immediately, and affects it in a way that
night does not duplicate. The same simple method is
effective with many related animals with compound eyes.

Abrupt cessation of messages from the eyes to the brain appears to block the timing mechanism. But how?

Perhaps the most spectacular halt in an insect's activity is the one called during development, aiding the animal to survive the winter where cold weather comes regularly. It is as though the creature had a calendar as well as a clock inside its body. Because grasshopper eggs and moth pupae showing this behavior are plentiful, scientists have been able to look into the workings of the system. In each case, the insect's brain seems to overcome the pause in development, as soon as the weather becomes warm after a few weeks of near-freezing temperatures.

Even an excised brain from a pupa that has been suitably chilled, if implanted into an untreated pupa in early autumn, will serve as an alarm clock, rousing the insect into proceeding with development. Evidently, after the cold treatment, the brain produces hormones that overcome the inhibitory effect of glands elsewhere in the body. Only then can the moth pupa complete the transformations that convert the resources of a caterpillar into the potentialities of an adult moth, ready to emerge and find a mate. Similar hormonal control centers interrupt development of a grasshopper egg until spring, then let it continue toward the day of emergence of an immature grasshopper.

The grasshopper egg and the moth pupa are clearly controlled by chemical compounds. Their calendar mechanisms seem to correspond to whatever it is that makes a seed pause in the midst of its development and wait for spring. But in this calendar we can see a difference from the rhythms that follow sun and tides and phases of the moon. From the internal calendar we have recently glimpsed something new in the amazing complexity of inheritance: a blend of birth and death in cells, and the genetic basis for the final countdown on cells doomed to die.

The egg, the pupa and the seed are all readying themselves for transformations to maturity, changes so tremendous they seem to be miracles. Each step of the maturation process, however, depends upon the release of a few more inherited directions from the nucleus of every cell. The hormones that induce these living things to become dormant before winter or dry season comes must serve to prevent emergence of these new directions from the nuclear centers. They restrain further maturation until a later time, when the season will be right. They preserve youth, in fact, just as though putting it in cold storage.

We might exclaim at the wonder hormone, the youth preserver, if it were not for something else that this chemical compound locks up in the nucleus as though it were Pandora's box. For insects at least, and probably for man as well, the emergence of the final directions for bringing the animal to full maturity is accompanied by the appearance of degenerative changes. Death too is in those last directions. The inheritance of an animal of almost any kind includes the chemical guidance each cell must follow for youthful growth, for maturity, and for senile decay as well. The moon no sooner reaches full than it wanes again. With life, the next waxing has its parallel in a new generation rather than in resurrection of the old.

This overlapping of youth, maturity and age is completely in accord with a philosophic emphasis on the continuous nature of time. Life is the finest example of eternal change and constant motion, of the flow of time, and the transitory nature of everything our senses bring to our attention. Each sense, as we use it to catch impressions from the surrounding world, is like a finger plucking a series of notes, contributing to an endless symphony. The players change, each one having played his part. But the music goes on. Time and space are the purest concepts we have found in all our wondering about the universe.

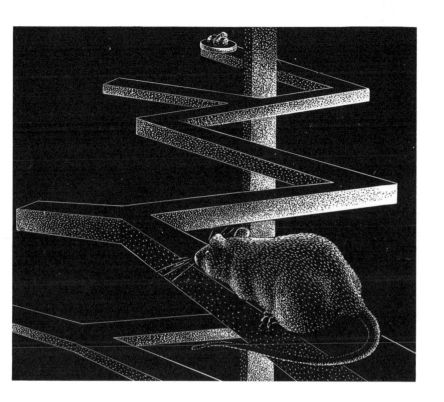

15. *Habitual Movements*

A RABBIT racing for home along a crooked path in the black of night and a small boy playing "by heart" a piece of music at a recital have more in common than merely the relief of reaching the goal at the end. Both of them are relying upon muscular movements in rapid succession, following a pattern etched by long practice into barely conscious parts of the nervous system. Both are depending upon their kinesthetic sense rather than on any visualization of the path or of the page of music.

Kinesthesis is often called "muscle sense," although actually its sense organs are located in the tendons and joint membranes as well as in the muscles themselves.

187

From all of these centers we receive a continuous supply of information about the movements we make and the pressures or tensions produced in various parts of the body. To a surprising extent we rely upon kinesthetic sense in moving about in familiar surroundings—and realize this chiefly when someone relocates a heavy piece of furniture or a doorway without telling us about it. Then we are likely to bump ourselves. Yet, until less than a century ago, no one considered our sensitivity to motion important enough even to give it a name.

Other animals seem at least as prone as we to ignore the more obvious senses at times, and to rely upon kinesthetic habits. We'll long remember a mother streamer-tailed hummingbird in the Hope River Valley of Jamaica, where we were trying to make a motion-picture record of the growth of her nestlings from the hatching to the flying stage. Day after day, just when she was about to land on the nest or was feeding her youngsters, a sudden breeze would displace the branch upon which the lichen-clad and demitasse-sized nest held securely. No close-up photography was possible under these circumstances. We decided to tether the branch to some stones. But the wind still caused the nest to bob up and down faster than the camera could follow, until we tightened the cords and produced tension in the branch greater than the force of the wind. Then we discovered that the mother bird flew to her young by kinesthetic sense rather than by vision. She buzzed to wherever the free branch would have held her nest, and tried to alight even though the nest itself was in plain sight about six inches lower and to one side. Since we always released the branch before leaving for the day, she never did learn to land gracefully on the nest in our chosen firm position!

No doubt displacements of this kind occur naturally. A strong wind may hurl a nest with its eggs unharmed to the ground. Rarely does the parent continue with it in the new location. Are habitual movements merely insufficient to bring bird and nest together again?

Kinesthetic sense, coupled with visual awareness of landmarks near by, provides many animals with most of the basis for near-automatic return to places of importance to them. The sea bird reaches her eggs camouflaged on the open beach by cues of this kind, and rarely needs to consider the details of the situation. Some animal may steal the eggs, but only a person is likely to shift them two feet to one side. A gull's eggs need not be moved far, in fact, before they become something to eat rather than possessions to be incubated. Similarly, honeybees coming to the hive may buzz in confusion for several minutes where the doorway previously was, before exploring on other sides of the box, if the beekeeper has rotated it during the insects' absence.

Despite the greater mental flexibility contributed by a larger cerebrum, most mammals also rely heavily upon kinesthetic sense. Scientists studying captive bats find that, after these dexterous fliers have learned their way around in a room—finding all the obstacles by echolocation, they will blunder repeatedly into a partition extending halfway across the room, whenever it is slid to a new position. By using suitable microphones and transducing equipment, the bats can be shown to be still uttering their ultrasonic chirps while flying. Echoes must be bouncing back abundantly from the partition in its new site. Yet the bats are inattentive, or "can't believe their own ears." They show this until they have freshly prospected the room for obstructions. Reliance upon kinesthetic habit appears to explain why, when a mine shaft harboring bats is provided with a new entrance door, hundreds of them may crash fatally into the barrier the first evening it is in place. Collisions between migrating bats and tall buildings or radio towers could have the same basis. Perhaps only inattentive bats pay with their lives for neglecting to listen as they fly.

If our own eyes and ears were not so helpful as we find our way about, we would rely more upon memory and kinesthetic sense. The Russian psychiatrists B. N. Klosovsky and E. N. Kosmarskaya proved how adequate this awareness can be, when coupled with experiences through touch. They deprived seventeen puppies only three weeks old of their senses of smell, vision, hearing and equilibration through organs in the inner ears. At first the pups slept most of the time, although they awakened independently

when hungry or to eliminate wastes. Later, their periods of
wakefulness lengthened and they began to show play
movements. Although food could give them no odors—
only tastes—and they could not see what they were eating,
their choice of food did not differ from that of normal
pups. The deprived animals grew well, in fact. They learned
their way about and moved neither more carefully nor
clumsily than pups able to see, smell, hear and use sense
organs of the inner ears.

Closer home, Dr. Lester Aronson of the American
Museum of Natural History looked into the routine behavior of the two-inch goby fishes that are so common in
tide pools among the coral reefs along shores of the
Bahamas and West Indies. The little gobies rely for survival
chiefly upon the almost-perfect match between their body
coloring and that of the sandy bottom in the tide pools.
They gain too from their ability to hide under loose fragments or in the tunnels of various burrowing animals.
However, if the gobies are pursued, they usually leap over
the rim of the pool and almost invariably land safely in
neighboring water—often in the direction of deep channels
through which the tide is running. Dr. Aronson wondered
how they knew which way to jump, for it is impossible
under ordinary conditions for the fish to see the next pool
before leaping. He checked whether they orient in relation
to a low place in the rim of the pool, or to the position of
the sun or shadows cast by it, or to the direction from
which vibrations of surf might come. None of these seems
a plausible explanation. Neither does trial-and-error learning. The only alternative seems to be that, in swimming
over the pools at high tide, the gobies train their kinesthetic sense to match the shape of the bottom in the area
around their home pool. From this they might gain the
orientation needed when they are locked in the pools at
low tide. Instead of swimming over familiar ridges, they
merely jump.

It is no great stretch of the imagination to relate a West
Indian goby fish learning the channels in its tidal areas to
a Syrian hamster discovering the sequence of turns that
lead to food on an elevated maze in the psychology
laboratory. If anything, the hamster's problem may be

easier: eight steps and a left turn, three more and a right, six steps to another right, then repeat with eight steps to the next left—and so on. The principal difference lies in the ease with which the hamster can be tested during its rapid learning process. But what is tested? Is it kinesthetic sense alone, or memory alone, or a combination of the two? Should hunger, or nearness to the reward, improve memory, as it does the hamster's performance? Or does reliance upon kinesthetic sense merely become more important to the hamster under these conditions?

We may wonder how much our own muscular co-ordination depends upon the state of our nutrition. If the hamster, when eager for food, uses its muscles more skillfully in running the maze, perhaps the best flint arrowheads were chipped by lean and hungry men, who thereby became dangerous. Some have claimed that the skill of the arrowhead maker survives today in the skill of a dentist working on a cavity in a tooth. Is the most expert modern dentistry done just before lunch time?

We now have reason to inquire whether the Latin custom of a noonday siesta and a late dinner at night may not confer real benefits in the quality of dexterous work. Perhaps we gain unconsciously by scheduling musical programs in the late afternoon or well after the dinner hour, and follow—rather than precede—them by a formal tea with refreshments. The musician's hands or lips upon an instrument and a typist's fingers on the keyboard in an office conceivably make fewer errors when the stomach is ready for a meal. It might be important to know how closely kinesthetic sense and hunger are linked in our everyday performanee!

Both kinesthetic sense and memory are served by adjoining parts of the brain—the cerebrum. No one has yet untangled their complex interconnections. Nor is any wholly satisfactory explanation available for the miracle of memory, although a number of intriguing ideas have been offered. One hurdle in any theory is the enormous capacity of the system for recalling details. Some tests of perception suggest that the human brain sums up a new picture of the outside world every tenth of a second in each waking day. During that tenth of a second it can appreciate perhaps a thousand bits of information from the sense organs. In seventy years, the brain might store 15,000,000,000 such items—a number a thousand times greater than the total of nerve cells in the body. Clearly, each cell must be able to keep track of more than one bit of information and yield it upon demand.

Even such simple differences as a right turn or a left turn require time to become fixed in the memory. During the interval between an event and its fixation, the memory of it can be erased. Hamsters, learning to thread a maze, perform somewhat more poorly if they are given an electric shock one hour after each test run. They forget completely if the shock comes one minute after they have reached the reward. A shock at four hours after a successful run, however, has no effect upon learning. By then the memory of the route has been fixed, and the hamster will run the correct path with less hesitation and fewer mistakes the next time it has a chance to take the elevated highway to its dinner.

It is tempting to conclude that, as messages pass along the nervous pathways from sense organs to the brain, they leave electrostatic charges at distinctive sites. These charges seem to slowly induce local changes of a more permanent nature. When we do the same thing again, the electrostatic charge or the local change would be reinforced, strengthening the memory of the event. Is this the way we train our nervous system until we can lift a hand to just the right height at exactly the proper time to seize a doorknob in the dark as we sleepily wend the familiar route from bed to bathroom? Is this what keeps a rabbit from colliding with a tree as it twists and turns to elude a fox on home territory at night?

Each spring, when a house wren decides to build a nest in the empty gourd we hang on a tree just outside the study window, we marvel at the way the bird instinctively uses kinesthetic sense. She scavenges among the larch branches and under the elms for twigs of a size and weight matching her kinesthetic criteria. She brings each one to the inch-wide doorway to the gourd and stands on the little perch provided while she nibbles her beak along toward the end of the twig. Then she tries to enter the doorway with it. If it catches crosswise, she hauls back and nibbles again toward the same or the opposite end. At least a quarter of the time, she goes too far and loses the twig to gravity. Invariably she goes in anyway—as though she had something to add to the tangle inside. Never have we seen her dive to the ground after the twig she dropped, as a chickadee will do with a seed. No more than three in each four of her tries based on instinct and kinesthetic sense actually contribute toward the nest.

We think of our own kinesthetic sense as something we can use more intelligently. As a child becomes more adept on the piano keyboard, we expect signs of musicianship to develop. Beyond mastery of the finger movements should come a critical awareness (and deliberate adjustment) of the sounds produced, to get "feeling" and "excitement" into the music. We expect the typist to do more with her nimble fingers than merely transcribe dictation to the keyboard. She should produce a page that is both letter-perfect and balanced as to margins—as attractive as it can be. Her speed may never reach that of the typewriter repair man who sits down at every machine and taps out the same test sentence: "9876543210-a brown fox jumps quickly over the lazy dog." But he isn't testing his kinesthetic sense, even though he relies upon it. He has gone beyond, and types this sentence because it makes use of every numeral and letter of the alphabet, letting him examine the machine's performance with a critical eye.

A considerable part of man's recent success in modifying his environment arises from his skill at using tools. Largely this is a measure of his ability to develop, through deliberate practice, the semi-automatic movements controlled by kinesthetic sense that make each tool an extension of his hand and eye and brain. The master driver of an automobile has become unaware of the steering wheel and the pedals for brake and throttle. His hands and feet make semi-automatic movements that keep the car in relation to other traffic as though its steel and chrome were extensions of his own living body. His vehicle may be a giant tractor-trailer truck, but his handling of it is barely different from the self-awareness a bull elk must show while choosing a route through forest tangles that could catch on uptined antlers. And when, at the end of a cross-country run, the truck driver transfers his skills to a compact passenger car, he adjusts his concept of size just as the elk must do during the annual cycle of growth and shedding of another paired rack of antlers.

Kinesthetic sense is a part of self-awareness we often overlook. Much of it, in fact, eludes any conscious investigation. If we stop to think how we manage something, suddenly we lose our hard-won ability. We are like the centipede in the story, unable to run when asked "which leg goes after which?" How can we make better use of this mysterious inner sense of co-ordination? For a sense we have been slow to recognize, we do amazingly well with it. The more we understand it, the more likely we are to benefit from further applications.

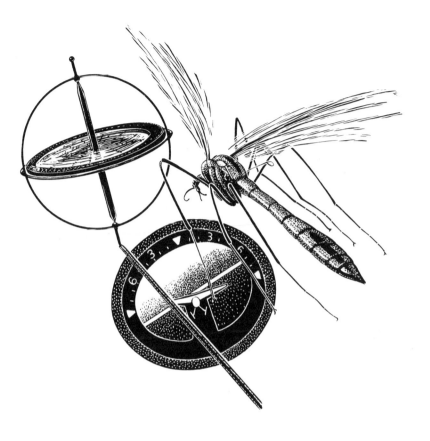

16. *Which Side Is Up?*

WHEN WE watch a toddler trying to co-ordinate his legs and supple spine in remaining upright, do we recall the intense concentration we applied to this same challenge between our ages of thirteen and thirty months? We needed years of practice before we could walk holding a glassful of water without spilling any. At first we managed by clutching it in both hands and watching it fixedly—letting our feet find their way as best they could. Later on, we needed the same profound application to the chore of walking with a shallow bowl full of soup. Do we remember these early difficulties when we see a waitress hurry with several dishes balanced on one arm, down the narrow aisle left by customers at close-set tables? Or the waiter watching her, holding a whole trayful of filled soup bowls nonchalantly backhand above his shoulder?

If we think at all about these skills, we are likely to conclude that our improvement was in muscular control linked to kinesthetic sense. We had to remain upright, and then detect any slight shift in weight as the liquid flowed toward one side of the container—in time to adjust muscular tensions, keeping the dish level. An acrobat performing in the circus act on a stretched wire is making comparable demands on his nervous system. But how far are these skills dependent upon the sense organs in our muscles, tendons and joints? Can we manage these balancing feats in complete darkness or with eyes closed? As we learned in childhood, our eyes can give us faster warning than our kinesthetic receptors whenever we (or things we carry) vary from attitudes of precarious stability.

Most of us, as children, experimented with our sensory adjustments in relation to gravity, and discovered other receptor systems in our heads. We stood on the lawn with arms outstretched and whirled like dervishes until we could remain upright no more. Our limbs were willing, and our eyes cleared before we could stand again without falling. But we proved to ourselves that our hard-won muscular co-ordination and our ability to correct our posture through visual cues could temporarily be nullified. All we had to do was overstimulate what the great American psychologist and philosopher William James called the "spirit levels" of the body. In each inner ear we have a set of three, as well as a little sensory sac containing tiny crystals of lime suspended close to receptor cells in fluid. These are our inbuilt equivalents of the electric turn-and-bank indicator a pilot finds so essential on the instrument panel of his modern airplane.

Our "spirit levels" are affected only by changes in position or changes in rate of movement. The fluid filling these semicircular canals must be shifted by a change to induce a sensation, and the response vanishes in less than half a minute after the change ends. However, the special sensory sacs connected to the canals respond to our physical atti-tude while we are stationary or moving at a steady pace. So long as these parts of our inner ear are intact and our kinesthetic sense is keen, we should have no difficulty maintaining our upright posture in the dark, or even carry-ing an open container of liquid—once we have learned how to use these sense organs.

It is astonishing how long early training of the sense of balance can last. Many an oldster, who has not been on a bicycle since childhood and has no idea that he can remain upright on one again, finds on a dare that he can still ride easily. If, as a child, he learned to pedal along, guiding the bicycle without hands merely by slightly inclining his body, he discovers that this feat too comes back within a few minutes of fresh practice.

So broad is our unconscious dependence upon kines-thetic sense and the organs of balance in our inner ears that we seldom give thought to what impairment of these organs would mean to us. One comment by a former asso-ciate on a college campus led us to a partial realization of this. Upon arrival at a class after a particularly deep fall of snow had made the morning walk difficult, he remarked how much he wished campus dormitories had bathtubs as well as showers, for then he would not need to live in a rooming house farther from the college. We could see no connection in this until he explained that a childhood attack of poliomyelitis, from which he had seemingly re-covered, had left him with almost no kinesthetic sense in his legs. In a tub he was safe from falling, whereas in a shower he would surely topple if he got soap in his eyes or for any other reason was forced to shut them for a few seconds. Only with his eyes open was he able to stand or walk.

A considerable number of people are congenitally hand-icapped by defective inner ears. They are incurably deaf, yet most of them can be taught to talk as well as to lip-read. Usually they lack also the normal sensations from their organs of balance in the ears. They compensate by paying more attention to kinesthetic sense and to visual cues. They may even realize that they differ from other people in being immune to dizziness from being whirled about, and to motion sickness produced through excessive stimulation of a normal pair of inner ears. Their awareness of the importance of compensating senses is usually keen. If they go swimming, they must stay in shallow water or risk drowning because, without the kinesthetic cues from body weight unbuoyed by water, they have difficulty telling which is up and which down. Such people, if blind as well, are usually unable to maintain their balance for more than a second or two if asked to stand on one foot.

The airplane introduces new confusion for even normal people in knowing which side is up. Any change in direction, elevation or speed becomes a stimulus to the receptors of the inner ears. They produce sensations that can build up into insistent belief, often as an interpretation of what is happening that is contrary to what the flight instruments show. A pilot flying a long glide path on the approach to an airfield may encounter a dense cloud just as he lowers his flaps or his landing gear. The plane decelerates rapidly, and his inner ears tell him that he is either bending over or going into a dive. He knows he is not bending forward. If he ignores his instruments and "flies by the seat of his pants," he is likely to nose his plane up, slowing it still more, until it stalls and he crashes short of the airfield. His instruments would show that his angle of approach had not changed when the flaps or the wheels came down. They could tell him too that the nosing-up of the plane was causing a dangerous loss of airspeed, and help him reinterpret the "evidence" from his senses of balance.

As passengers we encountered the reverse sensation in clear daylight upon takeoff in a Paris-bound jet plane from the Rome airport. The Caravelle's acceleration as we left the airfield was so rapid that it pressed our bodies well back into the cushioned seats. As the plane continued to gain airspeed, our inner ears told us that we were tilted upward at an angle of almost forty-five degrees. Yet, through the window, we could see the ground below us— at no such steep angle. Should we believe our eyes or our ears?

Many of the decisions necessary in flying modern aircraft at speeds up to a mile per second must be made from readings of instruments that are faster-acting and more reliable than man's various organs of balance. Most of these devices gain their stability from swiftly spinning gyroscopes which retain their orientation in space—and hence in relation to the earth—despite changes in the airplane's direction, elevation or speed.

During level flight, an airplane's controls need so little adjustment that an automatic pilot, suitably gyrostabilized, can take over the routine. But in landing and at takeoff, so much must be done on the basis of skilled personal judgment that a pilot is extremely busy—to the point of distraction—with dials, gauges, knobs, switches and landmarks along the runway. Nervous circuits from his eyes, ears and fingers are fully loaded. Yet the human element may make the difference between safety and disaster if something should be overlooked at a critical moment. For this reason, engineers have sought to find separate avenues to the brain that could be meaningful, reducing rather than increasing the number of tasks for the pilot's eyes.

In England, during 1960, a new use was found for the periphery of the visual field, based upon a familiar feature of vision. While standing still we automatically and unconsciously correct any tendency to topple forward, back or to one side according to any movement we detect "out of the corners" of our eyes. To simulate this peripheral field, three striped horizontal cylinders were mounted in the airplane cockpit, one on each side of the pilot, and the third just above his line of sight through the windshield. When the cylinders are rotated, the spiral stripes appear to shift and give an illusion of longitudinal movement to which the pilot responds instinctively. At no time does he need to look at the cylinders or feel any distraction from the runway, his instruments and controls. The cylinders can be driven by servo-motors coupled to devices sensitive to diving, climbing or banking of the aircraft. The pilot need only adjust his controls in relation to the spiral patterns until they stop moving. Without having to think about it, he simultaneously eliminates any tendency of his plane to pitch or yaw from the planned attitude for landing or takeoff. Success with this visual aid seems likely to direct the attention of engineers to further uses for this instinctive and relatively unexplored means for maintaining our balance.

While swimming, walking or running, we have no need for instrumental aids. Our vision and our inner ears seldom play us tricks in these slower modes of travel. Corresponding organs serve the other vertebrate animals, with the intriguing exception of the jawless lampreys. These aquatic creatures have only two semicircular canals in each inner ear, but possess a pair of large liquid-filled sacs in which the cilia on lining cells create a constant double whirlpool. Whether the twin vortexes are the equivalent of gyroscopes remains to be proved. They could be distorted by changes in the animal's position, and might help it recover its equilibrium after being tossed about by rough water in the rivers to which lampreys come at breeding time.

The French physicist J. B. Léon Foucault, who made the first gyroscope and gave it its name a little more than a century ago, was interested chiefly in demonstrating the rotation of the earth. His most spectacular success in doing so was with a long pendulum hung in 1851 from the roof of the Panthéon in Paris. Following the physical laws discovered by Isaac Newton, the pendulum continued to swing in the same plane despite the fact that the floor of the Panthéon, and Paris, and the whole world rotated below it. The same principle applies to a rapidly vibrating tuning fork, or even the knob-tipped balancers that represent the second pair of wings on a true fly. So far, the vibrating stabilizers of these insects have been imitated only in engineering laboratories. Tomorrow some useful application to man's needs may be found for them. But then, sixty years passed between invention of the gyroscope and its first use in navigation. Sixty-eight years elapsed before gyrostabilized instruments were developed for aircraft, permitting "blind" flying for the first time in clouds, fog or darkness.

To level various kinds of stationary equipment, man uses some very simple instruments. Some of them contain a bubble or a floating ball which rises to the highest point against the roof of its transparent chamber. Others employ a metal sphere which rolls to the lowest possible location on a slightly concave floor. Both are counterparts of minute organs found in animals. Even single-celled creatures appear to gain cues as to up and down, relying upon oil droplets or other microscopic spheres inside the protoplasm. Soft jellyfishes have granule-containing organs around the rim of the umbrella-shaped body. Hard-shelled crabs gain the same information from grains of sand in special pockets concealed in the first joint of the smaller pair of feelers.

The leveling devices of animals are so varied that we are reminded of something a wise old naturalist used to tell us: "An animal generally gets along in whatever simple way its body will allow." In a pond the common water boatmen capture a bubble of air between the body and each antenna, and detect vertical directions according to the way the buoyant bubble presses against the antenna. Backswimmer insects in a pond use the same method, but choose to live inverted, back downward toward the bottom. Snails appear to take their cues from the direction in which the shell's weight pulls on the body. A newborn opossum or kangaroo is its own plumb bob as it laboriously hauls itself, by alternate action of the precociously developed front legs, up the mother's body to her pouch.

Such a large majority of animals show a strong preference for an orientation with back up and belly surface down that we look with some surprise at any other choice. Why should a backswimmer row about inverted, and even show in its coloration—pale on the under, back surface and dark on the upper, belly surface—that for a backswimmer this is right and proper? Why should the fairy shrimps that appear so briefly each spring in pools left by melting snow, or their relatives the brine shrimps in salt lakes of western states, rush about back downward with feathery legs beating the water above them? Apparently there is nothing disadvantageous in this orientation.

A good many kinds of animals that clearly distinguish up from down are like ourselves in matching their body positions to particular occupations. The old-time sailors aboard a vessel under sail were ready to lie prone on a yardarm and reef in the canvas below them. A modern automobile mechanic thinks nothing of working under a car while lying on his back. Similarly a sexton beetle that scampers along the ground on all six legs rolls over onto its back to push below a dead mouse, or to lift the mouse little by little toward a suitable place for burial several feet away. A horseshoe crab runs along the sea bottom with four pairs of legs making co-ordinated contact with the surface. But when it wants to swim, it raises the front edge of the convex body and performs a vertical 180-degree turn that heads the animal in the opposite direction, upside down, with its legs and gill-cover plates flapping to propel it. When the horseshoe crab stops swimming, it settles to the bottom in this inverted position, and uses the long tail spine to right itself.

Among the most unusual animals in the world are the two-toed and three-toed sloths of tropical America, which hang inverted with hook-shaped claws supporting them from horizontal branches. By day they seldom move, but at night they travel slowly from tree to tree, eating their favorite foliage. Occasionally a sloth descends to the ground and drags itself along to another clump of trees. Only at these times, and when so young that it clings to the fur of its mother's chest and abdomen, does it assume a position with back up and belly down.

Our own recognition of whether some object or animal is "right-side up" or inverted is initially a decision based on touch, and then secondarily a decision we can make from visual cues. That touch is fundamental can be shown by equipping a person during all waking hours for several days with a special set of prisms that allow the light approaching the left eye to go instead to the right, and conversely. Through the right eye the person so equipped sees the world upside down, from the vantage point of the left eye. With both eyes open and the head in the normal position, the whole scene is exactly as it would be for a person hanging by his heels with his head at the same height. At first, the upside-down world is very disturbing, and walking through it or trying to do anything with the hands while watching them—inverted—a real strain. Yet in four days the person so equipped sees nothing amiss. The brain has accepted the change, and manual dexterity is back to where it was before the test began—with full

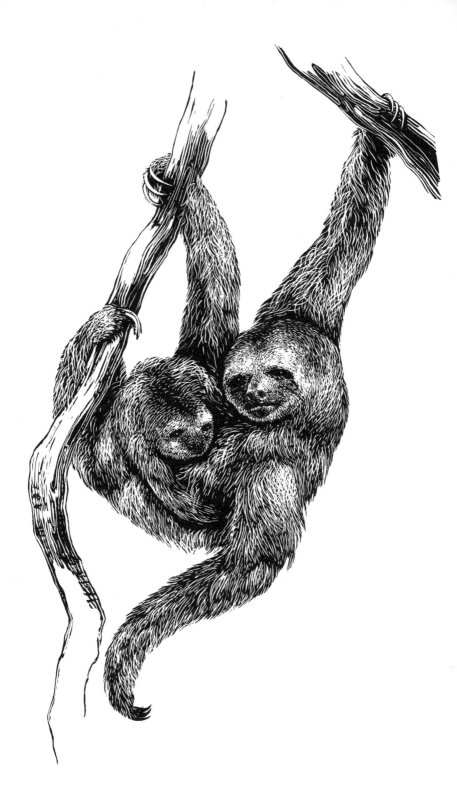

ability to guide the fingers by eye. But when the prism device is removed, the world in normal vision appears inverted again! Once more several days are needed to grow accustomed to the correspondence between what is seen and what can be felt with the fingers.

Seeing alone is not enough. If a person is equipped with spectacles that distort the visual field and is permitted to walk about, only a few hours of practice may be necessary before maneuvering is normal. But if the same person similarly equipped is wheeled about in a chair, no learning occurs. Similarly, if kittens are linked in a harness whenever they are in the light, letting one of them walk about while it can see while the other can merely see the same things without walking, their reactions develop an utterly different pattern. The unwalked kitten does not learn to avoid bumping into obstacles or falling off precipices, whereas the walking individual develops normally. Up and down, or other irregularities of the visual field, mean nothing to kitten or man until they have been experienced repeatedly as correlations between sight and touch.

Not all animals can learn to behave normally when their worlds are inverted or their organs of balance taken away. Some of them, such as the common periwinkle snails along the sea shore, show fixed behaviors in relation to gravity. These snails are attracted to light when inverted, and repelled by it when right side up. Similarly, an octopus that has been trained to distinguish between a horizontal and a vertical rectangle loses this ability permanently if its two organs of balance are surgically removed. Without its "spirit levels" it can no longer keep its eyes in any definite orientation. Failing this, its discrimination between similar shapes in relation to its surroundings vanishes.

Today man is posing for himself new problems for which the octopus is clearly not equipped. Every astronaut rocketing into space will be confronted with weightlessness. No longer will the tiny crystals of lime in the utricle of his inner ears or his kinesthetic sense organs bring him useful information as to direction. So long as his rate of progress or turn in any great curve remains constant, his semicircular canals will yield nothing his nervous system can interpret. He will be even more remote from reality than a pond strider on the surface film of a bucket of water being swung in a vertical circle around the ball-and-socket joint at a small boy's shoulder! More than ever, he will be a man "flying blind"—utterly dependent upon instruments to tell him where he is.

Except that his trip will be longer and his body enclosed in a protective capsule from which direct vision is likely to be extremely limited, the astronaut will be demonstrating the same courage and confidence in the handiwork of others that the parachutist needs when he steps through an open hatch to tumble earthward until his nylon canopy opens as it is supposed to do. But the parachutist can rely on gravity to tell him which side is up.

The astronaut will rely upon a cluster of gyroscopes to provide "inertial guidance" for his aircraft and its instruments beyond the reach of the earth's gravitational field. Would it comfort him to know that the largest insects that ever flew—with a wingspan of twenty-nine inches some 300 million years ago—and modern dragonflies as well, owe their dazzling aeronautical ability to an inertial-guidance system of the simplest kind? When a dragonfly's wonderful wing planes are tossed by an air current, the insect's massive head remains steady because of its inertia. The slender neck gives the body freedom to twist and turn. But any asymmetry with relation to the head is sensed through two little pads against which the head rubs whenever out of line. The pads are sense organs from which messages go to the wing muscles, leading them to adjust the flight and bring the body back into proper relation with the guiding head. And so the dragonfly darts along, gathering mosquitoes and gnats for food into the grasping basket of its bristly legs, stabilized by an ancient mechanism man has just begun to copy for his own far flights above the earth.

Evolution selected the dragonflies for survival from the Coal Age to the present. Aviation physiologists are trying to pick in advance those men most likely to succeed in outer space. From these practical studies are coming new understandings of the human mind.

Our perception of the upright is not a separate sense,

but one related intimately to the personality of the individual. Out of research over a decade at the Downstate Medical Center in New York has come recognition of astonishing differences among people in their preferred ways of perceiving. To some extent these differences may be inborn, for they are found well established at an early age and can be identified easily in the years from eight to thirteen. Later performance usually improves, but does not alter significantly the relative positions of the children within each group.

Many of the children and oldsters studied rely upon their eyes almost exclusively in identifying horizontal and vertical directions. They prefer to ignore cues from their inner ears, as well as from sense organs in the skin, muscles and tendons. These people usually show also a youthful dependence upon companions, and choose tasks they can perform in groups. Frequently they grew up in a home where parents were reluctant to delegate responsibilities, or severely restricted their activities.

Others studied are willing to discredit vision if it conflicts with sensory cues to their position in relation to gravity. These people tend to be independent by nature, often to the extent of being nonconformists. Generally they escaped early from parental ties, and broadened their own interests as though trying to contend effectively with more features in the environment. They commonly score higher on I.Q. tests because of greater skill in solving problems requiring the separation of simple patterns from a confusing complexity. They excel at using their senses in penetrating camouflage, although usually they show no special advantages in vocabulary, information or comprehension. It is simply that, in everything they do or the way they do it, the eye-independent people show a greater readiness to decide which way is up.

Each of us would like to know to which category we belong, and what effects this has upon our concepts of the world. How much are our skills influenced by inheritance and how much by our environment? Apparently our capacity for hanging a picture straight is linked to our ability in seeing a motionless bird in a bush. These discoveries emphasize the need for considering our sense in relation to total personality. The sensations we gain are not determined solely by the things sensed or by the limitations of our sense organs. Our brain too makes its contribution, and therein lies much of the uniqueness in each person's interpretation of the universe.

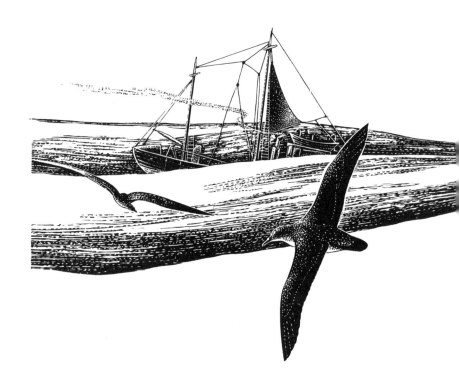

17. *Which Way to Turn?*

WHILE EXPLORING tide pools between sandbars near a dock in Pass-a-Grille, Florida, I (Lorus) met horseshoe crabs alive for the first time. I captured one and carried it to higher ground. I was ten years old. But when my interest in the creature began to wane, my parent insisted that I return it to the water. Then came the discovery: the horseshoe crab was already on its way to the sea. No matter how it was turned, or what slopes of sand were raised in its path, it unerringly shoved its armored body in the direction of the waves. How did it know its way?

Horseshoe crabs are not unique in showing a strong sense of direction. A host of different animals rely upon similar abilities. Yet until about a dozen years ago, the most widely accepted explanation was one suggested by Charles

Darwin, Alfred Russel Wallace and several others. According to these distinguished men, an animal retraces in reverse the route by which it is taken to a strange place. The method seemed so simple and logical that few people gave the matter further thought. Actually, animals take short cuts, as though they could triangulate and knew the direction to home base.

Claims for a more elaborate direction sense did not impress scientists so long as they came chiefly from pet owners. All such stories seemed to be fanciful, overdrawn or incomplete. Except in the way Darwin suggested, how could a dog or cat find its way home over unfamiliar territory from fifty or two hundred miles away? Animals have no road maps or compasses. Of course, no one knew what route the pets took between the moment of escape at some distant point and their arrival at the final destination. No fond owner would risk losing a pet in an experiment, or be willing to pay for a disinterested detective agency to shadow the animal for weeks if necessary, until it got home.

Animals other than pets tend to remain anonymous. Rarely can a person recognize them as individuals. Unless a chickadee has a numbered metal anklet, or a honeybee a distinctive pattern of colored paint daubed on her body, how can a person be sure when the same one is encountered a second time, or a third? Yet millions of birds were banded and recovered before anyone found a clear answer to the question: do migrating birds follow older, experienced members of the flock, or rely upon their own inner navigation sense?

The late Professor William Rowan of the University of Alberta released some young crows he had raised indoors, long after all other crows had left the Edmonton area and the ground was covered with winter snow. Several of the banded youngsters were recovered subsequently along the route they took—straight for Oklahoma, where Albertan crows of all ages go for the cold months. They were following a direction sense acquired in the egg. No parent birds or familiar landmarks could help them. They had no memory of past experiences.

Instinctive awareness of the correct direction for travel is stronger than any need to imitate. European bird banders discovered this after they replaced the eggs of West German storks with stork eggs from East Germany. The hatchlings received numbered bands and were watched until fall migration time. Then, when the West German foster parents set out for the Nile Valley by way of southern France, Gibraltar and the north coast of Africa, the fledglings raised from East German eggs went another way. They headed southeast and eventually joined flocks of East German storks, which migrate to the Nile Valley around the eastern end of the Mediterranean Sea through Greece and Asia Minor. Each individual bird separated at migration time from the common flock to travel on its own.

Similarly, no memory for turns or landmarks, and no parental guidance, can explain the ability of marked monarch butterflies from eastern Canada to fly as far as San Luis Potosí, some 1,870 miles distant in Mexico. Yet, after these insects have wintered in the warmer parts of America, enough of them return each spring to insure new broods of monarch butterflies from caterpillars on Canadian milkweed plants.

So astonishing are habits of this kind that they make us wonder about even the basic tenets of science. Are we correct in believing that sense organs are the sole channels of communication between an animal's nervous system and the outside world? Admittedly, this is an article of faith. Do the navigational and homing instincts of animals refute it, or is man merely insensitive to cues from the environment that are adequate stimuli for other animals? It is not enough for us to recognize that a direction sense is essential for birds, fishes, sea turtles, whales, bats and insects in migration, or for nonmigratory animals that return home reliably after being taken to unfamiliar territory. After realizing the extent of their ability, our own peace of mind almost demands that we find out how they know which way to turn.

The first step in this exploration for an unknown sense is to satisfy ourselves that animals do head in definite directions and follow this heading toward the final destination. Seldom can animals bearing distinctive bands be recovered often enough along the way to give a full account of their movements. To overcome this handicap, some biologists have learned to pilot a small airplane, and then have followed birds released in unfamiliar territory. The human fliers circled sufficiently high above the birds that the airplane did not seem to influence behavior. Pigeons and gannets did set out in the correct direction oftener than chance alone would explain. More recently, the designers of miniature electronic instruments for satellites have been called upon to devise lightweight radio transmitters that could be attached to birds or sea turtles. From radio messages emanating from these electronic cowbells, the exact whereabouts of the homing or migrating animal could be determined hour by hour. From records of the routes taken, the scientists still hope to discover the means of orientation.

Some people do seem to possess a vague sense of direction. They can go in one door of a department store and emerge through another on a different street in a strange city without becoming confused. They may drive at night along a winding street or take the proper turn out of a large traffic circle without hesitation or guiding signs, even when they have never before used the particular route. Yet, when asked how they do it, they have no answer. Other people usually distrust so vague a sense, especially when science has no acceptable explanation for it.

Confidence can be far greater when a magnetic compass is available. Today we tend to forget that only seven centuries have passed since the first loadstones and knowledge of how to use them to magnetize a compass needle came from China to Europe. Even the spelling *loadstone* (or *lodestone*) no longer shows that the piece of magnetite ore was a leadstone—leading the navigator in relation to the earth's magnetic lines of force. But do animals have compasses, or some other means for getting magnetic directions? Hundreds of pigeons have been flown with strong magnets fastened underneath their wings, in the belief that any magnetic sense they might have would be upset. The birds found their way to the home roost from many miles away in record time, despite the extra load. Comparable tests were published as recently as October, 1960, in the respected scientific journal *Nature*, showing that dead cockchafer beetles contain no permanently magnetic material such as could explain a claim made in 1957 that live cockchafers orient in relation to the earth's magnetic field. Without a compass how could the insects gain magnetic cues for their direction sense?

Equally recent discoveries that lampreys and fishes emit pulses of direct-current electricity to which their skins are sensitive may provide an answer to the questions concerning magnetic sensitivity in aquatic creatures. Perhaps the mud snail *Nassarius* relies upon something similar, for statistical studies of its creeping trails at different times of the solar day and lunar day suggested to Dr. Frank A. Brown, Jr., of Northwestern University that it orients in relation to "internal magnetic compass needles which in turn are hands of horizontal solar- and lunar-day 'clocks.'" The nature of the internal "compass needles" remains entirely unknown. That it may prove to be a widespread feature of living things is suggested by the almost simultaneous discovery that roots of peppergrass seedlings grow to align themselves in relation to geomagnetic forces.

If an animal could know its direction of travel and estimate its elapsed time and speed, it might use the equivalent of a human navigator's method of "dead reckoning." The late Werner Rüppell found that young hooded crows in Europe fitted this pattern. He captured nine hundred at Rossiten on the Baltic coast of East Prussia on spring migration, and banded them all. Four hundred he released immediately. The rest he took quickly to Flensburg, at the south end of the Danish peninsula, 465 miles due west. There he freed them in a region never visited by this kind of crow. As his banded birds were recaptured, he plotted the records on a map. Those released at Rossiten had all continued into their normal breeding areas east of the Baltic Sea. Those freed at Flensburg were caught in northeastern Denmark and in Sweden, all but one of them within an area resembling in form and dimensions the proper breeding territory—but displaced 465 miles westward. The hooded crows had continued in their normal migration direction for approximately the correct distance, and settled down. The only individuals that did not continue to shuttle back and forth each year, parallel to their relatives, were a few mature birds that had been captured by mistake. They seemingly recognized that their route was not taking them to the proper breeding region, and gradually worked back into their customary summering and wintering areas.

Even for dead reckoning, a navigating animal or man must know direction. Dr. G. V. T. Matthews of Cambridge University insists that pigeons and other birds get their cues from the sun, and that they can compensate for the varying angle toward the sun as each day progresses—low in the east at sunrise, high to the south at noon, and low in the west at sunset. According to his observations, a few minutes are sufficient for a pigeon to detect the arc the sun follows through the sky and for the bird to predict the arc to its highest point (due south). This is expecting a great deal of the bird's eye and brain, for the earth's rotation shifts the sun in the sky only about half the sun's apparent diameter each minute. Yet Dr. Matthews credits birds with far more than this ability to estimate accurately the sun's arc. He claims for them the equivalent of a sextant and a chronometer running on "home times." With these they can learn their geographical location anywhere on earth from the angular height of the sun at noon and the hour according to "home time" when it will reach this highest position for the day. The height will give the latitude, and the home time of noon the relative longitude of the place.

Anyone doubting that birds possess these instinctive skills is left with the difficult task of proposing an alternative, simpler explanation for the demonstrated ability of banded Manx shearwaters to fly separately over trackless seas from release points in America, for 3,050 miles in 12½ days to their own burrows on an island off the west coast of England. This performance required an average speed of better than ten miles per hour, day and night, or faster travel if the bird stopped at intervals to feed and rest. Each one must have sensed where home was in relation to America, even though Manx shearwaters never normally venture so far from the Isle of Man.

The sun is so conspicuous a skymark that no one doubts a bird's ability to see it. Our only hesitation is in accepting the flier's suggested talent for using the sun's position and arc in so sophisticated a way. Only a navigational instrument of considerable complexity will allow a human flier to adjust his travel heading automatically in relation to the sun as it follows its regular path from east to west. To use the moon, when it is visible at night, in a corresponding fashion—as has been claimed for birds migrating after sunset—would require reference to a lunar clock with a 24.8-hour day—measured from moonrise to moonrise.

Birds do migrate by moonlight. They also travel under the stars, with no moon, but seldom start out in cloudy or foggy weather. Could it be that these fliers are instinctively alert to the major constellations and can direct their flight by celestial navigation? Dr. E. G. F. Sauer of Freiburg, Germany, raised some night-migrating warblers in confinement, where they could get no glimpse of the heavens, to the age at which they normally would have begun their southward flights to wintering areas. In a closed box he took the fledglings to the planetarium in Bremen and uncovered their cage only after the dome above was illuminated solely by the projected replica of the major stars. Promptly the warblers adjusted their position in the cage to face in the direction their parents were already flying. While the caged birds were covered once more, the attendant rotated the imitation sky until constellations that should have been to the south were to the west instead. Upon removal of the cover, the birds adjusted their resting positions ninety degrees and again faced the southern stars. Nor did they alter their heading when the planetarium machinery was set in motion, slowly shifting the star pattern as it would appear to do through the earth's rotation. Actual directions meant nothing to them; they were navigating from celestial cues.

Even an electric lamp bulb shifted smoothly through an arc the sun might follow is enough guidance for a caged bird to turn and face the direction it would fly if free. Fishes too, despite their distorted view of the world above the water film, show that the sun and stars can provide the basis for accurate navigation. For a salmon, thousands of miles out in the Pacific, to remember for several years the angular elevation of the sun in the estuary of its home

river along the American coast, and to relate this to its
internal clock still running accurately on home time, impresses us far more than for the same fish to recall the
exact flavor of the tributary in which it hatched. From the
depths of our own minds we can recall an odor or a taste
never encountered between childhood and old age. We may
even remember the circumstances under which the fragrance was first met. Why are we reluctant to credit a fish
with sensitivities that have never been of comparable importance to mankind? Or a bird? Or a salamander?

Generally we try to oversimplify nature. We expect one
explanation to suffice, as a sort of universal truth. If a
pigeon, a shearwater and a salmon use cues from the sun
in their directional sense, we look for this same system in
all other kinds of life able to migrate or to find the way
home. Yet landmarks are highly important to some animals, as they are also to us. Possibly an abalone snail uses
some underwater equivalent of landmarks when it leaves
its daytime resting spot to feed elsewhere in darkness,
only to return before dawn to its homesite. At present, we
lack information on the navigational aids important to
various kinds of animals. But almost certainly they include
nearly every sensory stimulus to which life responds.

A few years ago, Professor V. C. Twitty of Stanford
University realized that he did not know whether the
salamanders whose embryos he had been studying lived
more than a year or two, or if they regarded as home the
particular stream along which they mated and laid their
eggs. To learn the answers, he marked distinctively 262
salamanders from a single pool and released them there
again at once. Year after year he caught and examined
every salamander he could find along the stream. Each
time he found a marked individual, he tallied it, marked it
again freshly, and released it wherever he found it. Only a
part of the marked population came to the stream in any
given year; in the seventh year, 32 per cent returned. But
many of them had not come for a year or two previously,
and did not return in the eighth year. Salamanders lived
a surprisingly long time; far more than 32 per cent must
be surviving.

Between breeding seasons, every one of these salamanders left the water. The population distributed itself over the adjacent mountainsides, and hid underground during the dry summer months. Yet almost without exception, whenever a marked salamander returned to the stream, it was faithful to the original pool.

Professor Twitty decided to relocate some distinctively marked salamanders to see if they could find their way back to the place where he had originally found them. Of nearly a thousand he transplanted to another stream three miles away, eighteen managed in the third year to get home. They had surmounted a ridge more than a thousand feet above the stream level to reach the original pool. How did they find their way?

Visual clues seem ruled out. Salamanders deprived permanently of their eyes reach their own breeding pools overland from a mile away. Touch is not necessary. In a star-shaped horizontal pen floored with plastic sheeting, they crawl slowly in the correct direction. Tilting the surface they rest on has no obvious effect. Apparently salamanders do not "feel their way home." Odor still is a possible sensory avenue for navigational guidance. Yet how could a salamander smell something distinctive about its own pool from three miles away and the other side of a ridge? As Professor Twitty "told the chaplain at Stanford, if it proves not to be a question of odor, then the whole problem really lies more in his realm" than in the Zoology Department. He will "gladly assign it to one of his theology majors."

Some such idea may have crossed the mind of the Italian entomologist F. Santschi in the second decade of this century, as he tried to account for the ability of North African ants to return to the nest. By erecting a high fence around an ant he prevented it from seeing any landmarks. With an opaque disk he shadowed the ant, concealing the sun's direction. And still the ant took the correct turns to hurry home. Santschi concluded that ants could see the stars and steer by them, even by day when to man's eyes the sky seemed uniformly blue.

Far more surprising was the explanation uncovered in 1949 by the master experimenter, Professor Karl von Frisch of Munich. He was seeking to discover how domestic honeybees communicated within the hive. How could a worker, freshly back from finding a source of sugar water, tell a dozen other bees exactly how far to fly and in which direction? Through a red pane of glass in the side of a hive, von Frisch watched returning bees that he had marked distinctively. They performed special little dances on the vertical honeycomb, while other workers crowded close. Whenever a bee from a feeder ten yards from the hive was dancing, she followed a circular pattern—always reversing her direction regularly at the same place in the circle. Any bee from a feeder a thousand yards distant performed a figure-of-eight dance, looping to the left around one circle, to the right around the other, with a tail-wagging run along the part of the pattern between the two circles. In these unlike dance patterns, von Frisch recognized how a worker showed the difference between "near" and "far." The far signal—the figure-of-eight dance—was faster too for food discovered at a hundred yards than for sugar water two miles away. At a hundred yards the dancer outlined about five complete patterns in each quarter of a minute, whereas at two miles, a single figure-of-eight was danced in this time.

Von Frisch saw that for sugar water far from the hive the "tail-wagging" run in the figure-of-eight dance varied in direction both with time of day and the direction from the hive to the food. Bees wagging as they ascended vertically on the honeycomb were indicating food to the east in early morning, to the south at noon, and to the west toward sunset. At noon, a returning worker full of sugar water from two hundred yards away wagged while descending the comb if the feeder was north of the hive, wagged while running horizontally to the left if the feeder was east of the hive, and performed her signal while running to the right if she had found food west of the hive. In every case, the angle between the tail-wagging run and the vertical on the honeycomb corresponded to the angle the worker bees should fly from the hive, using the sun as a skymark. The point of reversal in the "round dance" similarly gave the angle at the hive between food and sun. Herein lay the bee's means of communicating direction. Von Frisch described it as the "language" of the bees.

Like Santschi with his North African ants, von Frisch

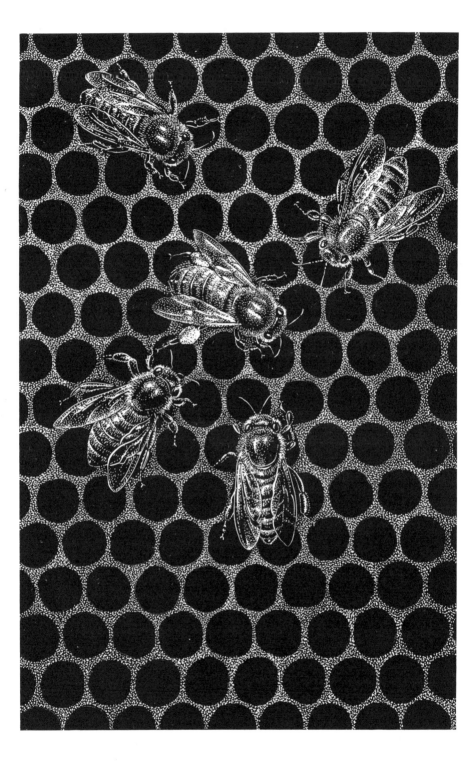

was puzzled to find that bees in Munich could still give and receive directions when the sun was hidden from sight by thick clouds, so long as a generous area of blue sky remained in view. Von Frisch had one advantage over Santschi: Polaroid sunglasses had been invented in the intervening years, and von Frisch was well aware that the seemingly uniform blue sky varies greatly in the angle of polarization shown by the scattered light reaching the observer's eye. Although the pattern is invisible to man without the aid of Polaroid materials or a Nicol prism, the compound eyes of insects might be detecting it. Using ingeniously simple tests with Polaroid sheeting, von Frisch proved that bees were indeed taking their cues from the polarized sky light as though it were a compass. With an internal "clock" compensating for the sun's apparent movement through the day, the insects use their "sky compass" for navigating successfully and for communicating direction within the darkness of the hive.

Recently, when tests were made with honeybees from Paris shipped by fast airplane to New York City, the insects were found to need only a little experience with the sun rising on a new schedule before they reset their internal "clocks" and began foraging on New World time. New York bees shipped to Paris soon made a similar adjustment. But when bees are shipped from the Northern Hemisphere to the Southern, they seem unable to learn their way about. The sun compass is reversed in the Southern Hemisphere, with the sun to the north at noon! Apiarists are finding that the ability of these insects to compensate for the sun's apparent movements east to west is inherited, with one mutation useful north of the Equator and its converse needed in the Southern Hemisphere.

If the compound eye is particularly well adapted for detection of the sky's planes of polarization, then sky compasses might be important to a really great variety of creatures. More than three quarters of the species in the animal kingdom have compound eyes. They are the insects on land and in fresh water, the horseshoe crabs that scavenge over the sandflats and into deeper coastal regions, and crustaceans with a multitude of habits. No longer need anyone doubt that the monarch butterflies migrating southwest from eastern Canada toward the Gulf of Mexico, and a separate population traveling due south from British Columbia to spend the winter in California, are navigating successfully in this way. A mutation giving an insect the wrong inherited sense of direction would likely be eliminated, leading to the present uniformity in each population. A mutant monarch in the northeastern corner of America, traveling south instead of southwest parallel to the sloping Atlantic coast, could have been ancestral to those nonmigrating monarchs now found in the West Indies. A mutant in the northwestern corner of America, following a southwesterly course instead of a straight south route, could have reached New Zealand and started a fresh colony "down under"—as happened toward the end of the nineteenth century.

In the years since Santschi puzzled over his ants and a child tried to confuse horseshoe crabs on their way back to the tide pools at Pass-a-Grille, those speculations have become respectable. A clear parallel to the horseshoe crab's direction sense has been discovered in another creature of sandy beaches. The sandhopper *Talitrus* along the Adriatic side of the Italian peninsula will automatically turn east and scurry toward salt water if taken inland. Near Naples or any shore facing Corsica and Sardinia, the sandhoppers go west toward Tyrrhenian safety. If a Neapolitan sandhopper is transported to the Adriatic coast, it still turns west—away from the sea and toward mountains it could never cross. In the wrong place, its inherited direction sense is disastrous. But so long as each population remains within its normal home territory, its sky compass proves valuable.

The Italians F. Papi and L. Pardi, who discovered these differences between east-coast and west-coast sandhoppers in their country, realized that night is the usual time for such crustaceans to be active on the beach. Astonishingly, the sandhoppers proved able to orient themselves correctly in moonlight. They wait until the moon rises and then set out on their travels in search of food. But can they guide themselves if the moon is hidden from them by some opaque object? Have they any counterpart of the celestial-navigation ability Santschi suggested? Must they even wait until moonrise to set their clocks each night?

No one was ever really satisfied that ants could see stars in the sky by day. It is equally implausible that sandhoppers can detect any polarization pattern in the night sky, or that they can see the constellations. Sandhoppers are about as blind as bats. Neither will respond to a pattern of imitation stars. Yet we know that insect-eating bats from northern latitudes include several kinds that migrate for hundreds or thousands of miles, even out over open ocean where they have no landmarks that would give a meaningful echo of an ultrasonic cry. How, then, by night, does a bat find its way over the ocean? Perhaps it relies upon sensory cues of which we are unaware—something no one has yet suspected.

The sky compass, like echolocation, is a discovery of recent years. We have every reason to expect further exciting revelations. Almost certainly they will include a further array of special senses showing animals—and possibly man too—which way to turn.

VI

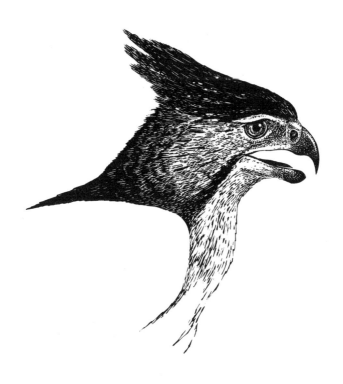

18. *Vision by Day*

RECENTLY WE watched, among the visitors to the observation gallery atop the Empire State Building, two boys vying with each other as to the makes and models of the various automobiles passing along the street below, at the bottom of the city's canyon. Even to tell a man from a woman among the pedestrians 1,250 feet lower than the observation gallery is a good test of eyesight. The small details of car design upon which the boys were basing their decisions reach the limit of human vision.

For most people, a cantaloupe at 1,250 feet would be the smallest object visible, and an apple or a mouse would be invisibly small. But to a hawk, chasing pigeons past the observation tower, a dime would be obvious on the sidewalk below. A mouse would be recognizable as food.

When using the best vision its eyes allow, a hawk has the equivalent of an eight-power magnifier with which to study the ground

Man has long been aware of the superior visual abilities of many birds. In the heyday of falconry, it was common practice to carry a small caged bird, such as a shrike, on the saddle horn. When the trained hawk was flown, it often rose too high for human eyes to follow it against the blue sky. The falconer could then tell where his tercel was by watching the antics of the caged shrike. The little bird instinctively feared the hawk and kept its head cocked to hold the falcon in view.

We too move our heads or our eyes to bring the image of objects interesting us to a small area of the eye where our most detailed vision is possible. When people twenty-one feet apart recognize one another by facial features alone, it is because each of the parties has brought the image of the other's face into this most discriminating part of the eye and there analyzed the minute picture (less than a fiftieth of an inch across) into some 283 separate areas in a search for familiar distinctions. This same infinitesimal portion of the eye's light-sensitive area is responsible also for the automatic reflexes with which we focus the image so sharply by adjusting our muscular control of the lens.

To make use of such refined analysis of the visual scene, the messages from this critical area of the eye are served by about eight hundred times as much area in the brain — a computer region where new visual experiences are compared with earlier ones in a search for meaning. The visual areas of the human cerebral cortex are divided almost equally between attending to the detailed central field and to keeping a general watch on the world through the large, vaguer remainder of the eye.

We rely so heavily upon past experience that we tend to see what we expect to see, and often overlook obvious features that would surprise us. Our eyes glance quickly from one tiny area to another, sampling the visual field, while our brain fills in the spaces between from memory. A few dark spots in a familiar pattern evoke the image of a whole cat — a particular one, perhaps belonging to a neighbor down the street. We fill in the missing outline of shadow

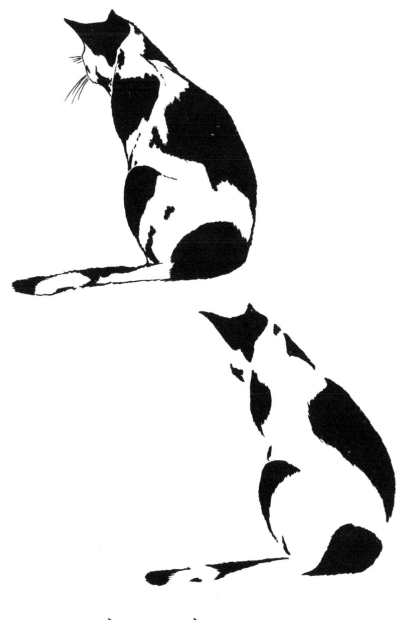

CAT

lettering, scarcely aware that the artist has provided only 50 per cent of each letter's outline. We can easily recognize the floral design on a china dish, find enough highlights to conclude that it is clean, estimate the size—whether tea plate or dinner—and fail to notice a nick in the rim until our fingers alert the brain. Then our eyes find the flaw.

The details the brain finds interesting or important seldom represent more than a small fraction of the sensations reported by the eyes. Moreover, one kind of creature differs enormously from another in the significance it attaches to specific visual experiences. This provides a challenge for mankind: to identify in other animals which features of the visual field actually lead to actions. In the European robin, it is a special shade of red matching the breast plumage of the male in nuptial garb. It releases a furious attack from the cock robin defending a particular piece of territory. No other simultaneous messages from the eyes seem to matter. It makes no difference whether the color is painted on the breast of a courtable female, or is only the dye in a tuft of wool impaled on a twig. The cock robin must drive it away or destroy it. Similarly, purple martins of both sexes will pursue gas-driven model airplanes with a deep purple fuselage and diagonal wing stripes, but ignore models of other colors.

We might expect that the wealth of visual detail spread before a gull or a buzzard patrolling a swatch of sky would preclude attention elsewhere. Yet the presence of distant dots in the sky, marking the soaring sites of neighboring birds, is at least as important as the seascape or landscape below. If any one of these neighbors descends, all of the surrounding patrol birds will move into the vacated sky space and search for the vanished one. With persistence they can join him below at a feast he has found.

Ornithologists, seeking to learn what features permit individual birds to be recognized by their fellows, have looked for details among a flock of domestic fowls. If an "inferior" bird in a well-established peck order within the chicken yard attacks a "superior" bird, a social error has been committed. Presumably the superior individual is no longer recognized. This occurs most frequently after alterations to the head (particularly the comb) and the neck of

the bird high in the peck order. Fowl, in fact, are discriminating to the point of clannishness. They will run
toward members of their own breed from as much as
140 feet away. At this distance a hen in side view produces
a visual image of the same size as that from a grain of
wheat at three feet—the farthest a hen will identify the
grain as food and run toward it.

How much a bird relies upon detail in the seed itself is
hard to show. On a cloudy day, chicks usually ignore seeds.
They will pass them by also in a room with such diffuse
lighting that the seeds cast no shadows. Even if the birds
have use of both eyes, they will often peck at seed-colored
areas marked on the floor if each imitation seed has a
black shadow painted at one side of it. The shadow seems
to be the feature upon which the bird judges size, distance
and shape. Lack of shadows may be the principal reason
why so many birds become inactive in dull weather.

Among birds and many other animals, a large proportion of these responses to details in the visual scene are
inherited. A newly hatched chick will ignore a duck flying
overhead, but react with obvious terror to a hawk. The
outline of a hawk and duck are not so different. The outstretched wings of each are comparable when gliding. The
long neck of the duck matches the long tail of the hawk,
and the short tail of the duck the closely-held head of the
hawk. The difference lies in which precedes—the long extension or the short. This is the chick's inborn cue. If a
black cardboard silhouette of a gliding bird is moved
across the chicken run on horizontal wires, and the long
extension precedes, the chicks are undisturbed—it's only
a duck. But if the long extension trails, they scatter and
hide—it's a hawk!

Chicks that have been hatched in darkness and not yet
fed are alert to small patterns the size of an edible seed.
Repeatedly they will peck at a spherical pellet of contrasting color behind a thin glass plate, clearly preferring it to a
flat disk or an angular three-dimensional pyramid of the
same size at an adjacent window. An innate preference is
evident. It makes us wonder how much human babies are
ready to discriminate at birth.

Infants are harder to test, for they seem to get bored and

doze off. Yet some, watched at Western Reserve University within two weeks of birth, showed significant differences in the length of time they would stare at circular patterns displayed in pairs. Disks marked boldly to suggest a human face received much more attention than disks of the same size with identical marks (representing eyes, brows, nose and mouth) in meaningless arrangement, or plain disks of any gray or color. Already—and perhaps from an inborn ability—the babies were attending to those features by which adults distinguish one another and judge mood. We could regard this as the beginning of social awareness. Apparently it improves rapidly as the child's eyes register finer detail. At one month, a baby needs any feature to be sixty times as coarse as an adult does to distinguish it. By six months, however, the child is aware of smaller objects, and already sees details only five times as coarse as the finest an adult can see.

Vision plays an important role both in the young's identification of the parent and in the parent's ability to recognize her own young. The newly hatched duckling, in fact, becomes "imprinted" by the first moving object it sees after emerging from the shell. The object may be a mother duck, or a decoy towed by a string, or a person, or even a motorcycle traveling slowly along. Whatever it is, the duckling forms a firm lifelong attachment and re-sists any substitution, however natural. Correspondingly, until a mother dog or cow or rat has had a chance to look carefully at her new offspring, she will accept a substitute even, in many instances, of quite a different kind.

Early visual impressions are generally important in influencing the later behavior of animals. The first three days appear to be critical for the migratory locusts of the Middle East and Africa. Any individual grasshopper that encounters no others of its kind during this period after emergence from the egg develops a permanent preference for solitude and shade—and generally avoids other locusts. Under crowded conditions, by contrast, the newly hatched grasshoppers form companionable aggregations. They tolerate the full sun and soon develop the habit of traveling in vast numbers to seek food in new locations, bringing ruin to man's crops. It is tempting to wonder whether

Thoreau would have preferred his own company so strongly had he been born in a modern hospital and spent his first few days in an air-conditioned room as a member of a close-ranked crib population. Is visible crowding at an early age turning mankind into a race of migratory 'hoppers?

Probably we communicate by eye with our fellows a great deal more than we realize Marcel Marceau and other professional pantomimists have spent a lifetime refining their art of bypassing verbal language, and conveying messages to audiences without regard for age or national cultures. Perhaps the universal idiom of the circus clown is older than any spoken word.

Slight movements and quick glances can often keep close companions in tune. These informative actions, although often overlooked. sometimes bridge normal barriers between unlike kinds of creatures. All of the horses and dogs credited popularly with the ability to count or spell have proved upon careful testing to be alert and responsive to trivial cues seen in their master's behavior. How much can a horse or dog learn from some other animal by similar attention to slight movements? Our physician insists that dogs communicate by eye, and that a visitor's dog will enter his living room without hesitation only if he blindfolds the springer spaniel at his feet by the fireplace. Does this prove that the strange dog receives a warning from the eyes of the physician's dog, or that the springer by the fire will, unless blindfolded, react to the arrival of the visitor's dog with some slight movement the newcomer detects?

For ourselves, as for every other kind of animal with eyes, identification of potential food ranks high among the uses for vision. Yet, as the eighteenth-century philosopher David Hume pointed out, "neither sense nor reason can ever inform us of those qualities which fit it for the nourishment and support of a human body." What is there about any food we have never tasted that tells us it is safe—let alone good—to eat? What features of yellow-banded black insects lead even an inexperienced European bee-eater bird to seize, wipe vigorously in a way that ruins any stinging mechanism present, and then take the insects as food?

What aspect of visual sense tells a toad when an insect is small enough to treat as prey and when of a size to release the toad's defensive behavior?

Visual cues of highly special types are linked to courtship, for only creatures with fairly good eyes court their mates. Yet the number of identifying features must be small. How otherwise could an orchid flower fool a male parasitic fly looking for a female of his kind? Some orchids apparently provide just those few critical cues and induce the insects to perform a false mating with the flower, pollinating it in the process.

In comparing the various roles of vision in mankind with those recognizable in other members of the animal kingdom, a great cleavage might be expected between the visual world of man and other animals with a backbone and the visual world of insects and crustaceans. Our eyes, as also those of the octopus, the cuttlefish and squids, are relatively soft. They are embedded in the body for protection, and have a single lens serving all the light-sensitive cells. If the photographic camera had not been invented independently, most of its principles could have been deduced from an eye of this kind. Animals with a camera-style eye, however, comprise less than 6 per cent of the species in the animal kingdom. The vast majority—more than 77 per cent—are insects and crustaceans with compound eyes like those of honeybees. A compound eye has a hard outer surface bulging from the body, and a separate lens for each dozen or so light-sensitive cells. How different is the world through an insect's eyes?

Each of the two bulging compound eyes on the head of a three-quarter-inch honeybee is composed of about four thousand slightly tapering tubular units fitted together like the seeds in a sycamore ball. Each unit, with its separate lens, is responsible for keeping the insect informed of any changes in the amount of light coming from some one small portion of the total field of view. An eye of this kind is particularly sensitive to movement, as pale or dark areas in the visual field affect one after another of the radially diverging units.

At its best, the bee's vision is much poorer than our worst. For an object to be visible to a bee, it must be relatively huge—one hundred times as large as for a person to see it. At the edge of the bee's visual field, it must be six thousand times as large. This seems almost incredible when one recalls the small flowers a bee seeks out. However, the paradox is easily explained. The bee does not see a single flower until very close to it. The angle subtended at the eye is the important feature. Since our eyes cannot focus on objects at very close range without a powerful lens to aid us, we tend to overlook the magnifying effect available to animals that do see things from a nearness of an inch or less.

Understanding how the insect sees the individual flower does not account for the bee's finding the blossom in the first place. This arises through its ability to detect movements. We often catch sight of a moving object "out of the corner of an eye." If it is a sparrow or an insect, the object is far too small to be seen in the extremities of our visual field—until it moves. Then its image shifts from one area of the light-sensitive retina to another, and our eyes report "something" without identifying it. We turn to look at it directly, and gain about sixty times as much detail in this way.

Similarly, if something moves in a bee's visual field, the event is reported to the tiny brain. It makes no difference whether the movement is due to a flower waving in the breeze or the bee flying past the flower. If the blossom affects one part of the compound eye after another at a reasonable rate, movement is reported. The bee comes down for a closer look.

An apple tree in full flower, surrounded by green grass or weeds, is an object a bee can see from a fair distance. The white of the tree contrasts well with the background. At closer range the insect may be able to tell that the flowers are in clusters, with green or dark areas between. If the blossom-bearing branches are agitated by the wind, they are far more attractive to honeybees than a tree sheltered from the breeze by a building. The former will be fuller of insects which have been flagged down by the extra movements of the white areas across their visual fields.

The bee's compound eyes are no more efficient, of course, than the nervous system to which they are connected. It is the combination of eye and brain that gives the flying insect its special sensitivity to movements. This gives it also an ability man has longed for ever since he developed aviation. But until he could workably imitate with electronic circuits the nervous system serving the compound eye, this important application remained beyond his grasp. Now engineers have devised for aircraft a ground-speed indicator patterned after an insect's eye. One unit is located in the nose of the plane, a second in the tail. Both units face the ground. Electronic circuits measure the time a pale or dark area on the ground takes to travel from the one limited field of view to the other. This information, when related automatically to the height of the plane above the terrain, yields a computed indication of miles per hour in terms of travel across a map.

Quite evidently insects use their compound eyes in just this way. If they encounter a headwind that is sweeping them backward as fast as they can fly or faster, they descend and settle until the breeze subsides. The pilot flying a ninety-mile-per-hour light aircraft in a ninety-mile-per-hour headwind might just as well land too, for he is actually standing still above the landscape. He is wasting his gasoline, chopping the wind. Yet until the compound eye was imitated in a ground-speed indicator, the pilot had little to go by except his air speed, telling him that his plane was traveling some number of miles per hour in relation to the air passing his wing tips. A knowledge of what his airplane is doing in relation to the ground is far more meaningful when navigating a trip.

Motion of some kind seems essential for vision. The honeybee achieves it by flying over the landscape. The predator patiently waits for some other animal to move and reveal itself as prey. We supply our own movement by shifting our gaze. Minute rapid adjustments of the muscles controlling our eyes keep them quivering slightly, up and down, or sidewise. If special contact lenses are mounted on the eyeballs, holding constant the visual field wherever our eyes turn, the effect is startling. The colorful picture fades into a uniform nondescript brownish gray! Only by minutely shifting the visual image on the light-sensitive cells in the eye do we keep them from adjusting completely to whatever intensity of illumination strikes them. Otherwise they cease sending messages to the brain. Our inability to hold our eyes really steady is actually a gain.

Most animals seem to lack these very slight jittering movements of the eyes. Unless something moves in the visual field of a frog, essentially no messages travel from the eyes to the brain. Ordinarily its view of the world must be as blank as a clean blackboard. Any walking or preening insect, however, surely stands out as though vignetted.

So strict is the amphibian's demand for movement in detecting food that until 1960 any captive individuals were either allowed to fast, or given active insects and worms, or hand-fed with bits of meat waved slowly within reach. Then Connecticut psychologists Walter and Francis Kaess invented a sort of toad-o-mat in the form of an electrically rotated platform on the rim of which they placed bits of hamburger. Toads quickly learned to stand near the rim of this Lazy Susan and pick off the ground meat as it passed. Some toads even crept up on the rotating platform itself, and discriminated between the hamburger and its background even though toad and meat now revolved together. Probably the food did not blank out for the rotated toads because these animals make slight involuntary body movements as a jerky response to any continuous shifting of the whole visual field. Even these slight movements would keep the hamburger in view.

The richness of our visual scene is lost only if its pattern sweeps past our eyes at too great a pace. About ten distinct pictures per second seems to be the most we can sense separately. Even at this rate, successive patterns must be roughly similar if the mental image from them is not to blur. We fuse into a continuous action the sixteen pictures per second projected on a home-movie screen, and scarcely detect the thirty-two brief blackouts of the projection screen each second. At sixteen blackouts, however, or a slower rate of replacing each photograph with another, the flickering becomes objectionable. We can detect also the fluctuations in intensity of illumination from incandescent lamps run on twenty-five-cycle alternating current, such as was produced until recently at Niagara Falls. Lamps run on fifty-cycle or sixty-cycle current convince us that they are perfectly steady. Similarly, we never see the fast-moving dot from the electron beam in a television set as it bamboozles us into believing a picture is on the face of the tube. Unless we are too near the instrument, we even fuse together the whole pattern of parallel traces the dot travels in sequence.

In these respects we differ greatly from many of the animals with compound eyes. A housefly or a honeybee can distinguish between a steady light source and one flickering more than two hundred times a second. Apparently these creatures compensate through a spectacular temporal awareness of changes in the visual scene for their poor ability to distinguish separate spatial details. There can be no doubt that this talent for seeing separate patterns in sequence at high speed is important in a flying animal traveling at low levels between all manner of obstacles at a pace between five and ten miles per hour.

Strangely enough, more is known about what is meaningful to the eyes and brain of an insect seeing a pattern than about how we ourselves recognize the letters of the alphabet. Honeybees can be trained to come for drops of sugar water placed on horizontal panes of thin glass laid over coarse patterns—circles, triangles or rectangles. If fed repeatedly over a black disk, the bees will ignore open squares, X marks, or even black rings of the same diameter as the disk. Yet they cannot distinguish among black disks, black triangles and black squares of unlike size if all of these patterns have the same perimeter. An X and an outlined triangle will be confused if they have the identical number of inches of boundary between black and white.

The insect does not recognize shape as such, although it can associate food with a crude measure of a pattern's outline. This is the feature distinguishing a three-petaled flower from a five-petaled one of the same diameter. It accounts for the bee's ability to visit a single kind of flower repeatedly, then ignore those blossoms from which the petals have begun to drop.

With coarse patterns, an octopus or a land tortoise can be more discriminating than any creature with a compound eye. But so far no one has learned how these animals evaluate their visual scene. Perhaps their method might be refined and applied to a new marvel of electronic circuitry. If only a device could scan a filing card or the title page of a book and identify a roman A as being the same letter as an italic *A*, a script *a*, or a lower-case printed a, the machine might attend to the filing and retrieval of documents in a storehouse of written words. Some people are reluctant to see success in these endeavors. They fear that the engineers will bring us full circle in finding extensions and substitutes for human senses, by replacing man as well. Others see no danger, and are hopeful of real progress. All of these people wonder how man recognizes patterns, whether the seemingly simple ones of a phonetic alphabet, or the complex forms of Chinese ideograms. What will it require to build a machine that can serve as a librarian?

In nature, only an animal as big as an elephant, as strong as a black leopard, as trigger-touchy as a skunk or as wily as a crow can afford to let its body pattern show. Other creatures are safest or surest of a dinner when they disappear. Unfortunately for the preyed-upon, the predators usually have the best eyes and brains attuned to using visual cues. To elude them without flight requires both the courage to stay perfectly still and camouflage to make such inaction rewarding.

A considerable part of our success in unmasking the camouflage of animals lies in specific features of our vision. One of them is our awareness of the boundary between two gray areas that differ as little as one per cent in the amount of light they reflect. This gives us approximately five hundred shades of gray between white and black. On the other hand, a honeybee must have a 25 per cent difference between two shades of gray to be able to detect the boundary between them. As a result, its eyes can distinguish only about a dozen grays, plus black and white. The little fruit fly *Drosophila*, which has been used so extensively in the study of inheritance, has only three shades of gray in its visual range.

Related to this deficiency of grays in the vision of insects is their response to darkness. An insect that is active only in daytime believes that night is at hand if the illumination drops rapidly to a hundredth of the sunshine level. The insect may go to sleep promptly, as many brave souls know who have captured a bumblebee in hands cupped together around the buzzing insect when it backed from a flower. Try it! Don't be alarmed when the captive shrills a warning as it creeps around the closed surface of your palms. The sudden darkness overcomes its concern, and it quiets down with astonishing speed. Several seconds of direct sunlight are needed to awaken the sleeping bee again. During the twilight of solar eclipses almost the whole insect population goes to sleep.

Even when allowed an hour to grow accustomed to a darker place, the compound eye needs a thousandth of full illumination to see. We get along well with only a billionth. For this reason, if no other, daytime insects do not awaken with the birds, but stay quiet on their sleeping sites until the sun has cleared the horizon and filled the shadowed spots with light.

Ordinarily we give little thought to shades of gray. Juncoes and catbirds are gray. So are Maltese cats, beech bark and slate. But otherwise this is not a common shade among natural objects. Most things we see are blue, like sky or larkspur; or green, like chlorophyll; or yellow, like canaries and dandelions; or orange; or red. The grays to which our eyes respond are supplemented by an almost limitless range of colors. Only when we see these hues translated into grays in a "black-and-white" photograph or on a television screen do we encounter the world as most animals see it. At other times we use our color vision as an extra means for penetrating camouflage and finding meaningful contrasts in the visual scene.

Despite popular belief, there is nothing especially attractive about a red flag for a bull. Anything waving excites the animal. A white flag or cape would be far more visible to him, and hence more effective, because the bull is color-blind. So are the cow and horse, the dog and cat, the pig and sheep. None of them can be trained to go for a reward to a colored square of any hue, if it is placed at random in a checkerboard of grays from white to black. Of all the mammals, only man and some primates enjoy the luxury of color vision.

The exact details of color vision remain one of nature's best-kept secrets. Yellow, for example, is a sensation induced just as well by alternately flashing red and green light into one eye as by stimulating it with the "yellow" part of the spectrum. White is equally an interpretation of the brain, one that can be induced in many different ways in addition to the usual one—providing a mixture of wave lengths at suitable intensities to correspond to that in sunlight.

The day-active birds and most reptiles see color. So do all fishes that have been tested carefully. Frogs and salamanders apparently are color-blind. The use of red flannel to induce bullfrogs to snap at a hook on the end of a line is a fallacy like that of the bull and the red flag.

Bees show the magic ability to distinguish a color from any shade of gray. So do a number of crustaceans, the squid and the octopus. But this is not to say that they see colors as we do. In the case of the bee, at least, this is far from true.

Part of the difference in the colors an animal can see lies in the extent of its spectrum. One of the most convincing demonstrations on insects was performed a few years ago by the British entomologist, H. Eltringham. He caught several of the common butterflies known as Tortoise-shells, in the pattern of whose wings red is conspicuous. Using a clear red lacquer, he painted over their compound eyes, fitting them in this way with harmless red glasses. Then he let them free, and noted that they flew as well as usual. Apparently the Tortoise-shell can see in red light, which alone could pass through the red lacquer. When the same test was tried on the white butterfly known as the Large Cabbage, the insect flew aimlessly, with reactions like those of a blinded insect. These observations match the behavior of the two butterflies, since the Tortoise-shell visits red flowers, whereas the Large Cabbage rarely does so. Apparently it is unable to see them as more than black shadows.

Our own vision has its limits too, and the brain can do nothing directly to broaden the range of colors visible in a rainbow. Our limit at the violet end of the spectrum is imposed by the filter action of our slightly yellowish lenses, which absorb the ultraviolet. As we age, in fact, our lenses grow progressively yellower and filter out some of the violet too. Old painters seldom become aware of this, but their paintings rarely include true violet hues.

We have reason to be curious about the ultraviolet, for to a honeybee it is the most stimulating part of sunlight, as well as a distinctive color—different from violet-blue, blue-green, or greenish yellow. Objects that reflect ultraviolet are far brighter to most insects than objects that do not. We fail to see these differences, although we can use photographic film or television cameras sensitive to ultraviolet as a means to explore the world of insects in this part of the spectrum. Most things that reflect light visible to us also reflect some ultraviolet. A few provide surprises. The common yellow daisy, for example, absorbs ultraviolet except at the tips of the petals, which are intensely reflecting. In consequence, this flower is visible to insects as a halo of bright ultraviolet spots surrounding the central cone where the nectar and pollen wait.

Some insects too show strange features in ultraviolet. Both the male and female luna moth are a pastel green to our eyes. In the ultraviolet, however, she is a blonde and he a brunet. These differences must be visible to the moths whenever they see one another in daylight.

The moon, for which the luna moths are named, reflects almost no ultraviolet to the earth. Nor do animals more than an inch or so below the surface of lakes, rivers or the ocean encounter ultraviolet, for the top layer of water converts essentially all of it into heat.

Comparatively few creatures spend the daylight hours cruising at the surface, but some of these are fitted especially for seeing in both air and water. Divided compound eyes are the mark of the black whirligig beetles which spin and dart on the surface of ponds and lakes. One half of each whirligig eye faces into water and is always wet. The other half looks into air, and is located above the water line. The four-eyed fish of Central and South American rivers is similarly equipped for seeing in the dry world and the wet. Each eye has two pupils, and the fish swims at the surface with the upper pupils exposed to air, the lower ones looking into the water. In this way it is able to keep apprised of events all around it. The same lens serves both pupils, and the proportions of the eye are correct to allow clear vision through both of them simultaneously.

Ordinary fishes have a strange view of the world. Through the water they see objects on the bottom. Directly above them (and to all sides of vertical for an angle of exactly 48.8 degrees), they look through a window bounded by the horizon. This is due to the bending of light as it enters the water. Surrounding this window is a reflection of the bottom, poor or good depending upon how much the wind ruffles the water surface. So used to this queer field of view is any fish that it keeps close watch on every detail: the worm on a hook tethered by a line; the kingfisher hovering directly overhead; the snail creeping along the bottom. All are of importance.

Until the kingfisher dives in pursuing a minnow, it studies the situation with one eye—monocularly. Whichever eye is used, it brings the scene into focus through the combined light-bending action of the lens and of the curved cornea exposed through the bird's tears. So far, the kingfisher is doing as we would. When the bird dives, it is like us too in losing the focusing action of the cornea as soon as it is immersed in water. We find ourselves hopelessly farsighted under water unless we wear diving goggles or a mask, and keep our tear-wet corneas in air. The kingfisher has no such accessories. Instead, it makes use of the lopsided shape of its eyes, and directs its attention through them in a different direction—looking for the fish binocularly, straight ahead of the beak. In this direction the kingfisher's eyes have the right proportions for underwater vision and, with skill or luck, its quarry will be in view.

Only a few remarkable animals, such as seals and sea snakes, are like kingfishers in being fitted for keen vision in both air and water. Most are as limited as we. Fishes and the penguins that chase them have such strong focusing action in the lens of the eye that they need no help from the cornea to see while swimming. When a penguin emerges into air, however, the added focusing action of its cornea makes it pathetically nearsighted. It has difficulty distinguishing a stone from an egg at its own feet.

Perhaps the most important conclusion to which our eyes can lead us as we look about by day is that our particular combination of limitations and specializations in vision affords us almost boundless opportunities. It is true that we lack the periscopic vision of the rabbit and the woodcock, whose eyes are on opposite sides of the head and provide almost no binocular field. But by having our two eyes facing forward, we can use both of them at once in examining objects in our hands. This has contributed immeasurably to the development of manual dexterity, to invention of tools and to the whole evolution of civilized ways.

Today our tools include instruments of many kinds with which we extend our inherited visual abilities beyond the range of any other animal. With telescopes we probe toward the fringe of space, and with microscopes into an otherwise unsuspected world in miniature. It is hard to think back to times of lesser understanding. In our eagerness to expand our horizons we have changed our perceptual world itself and made it a new environment for mankind.

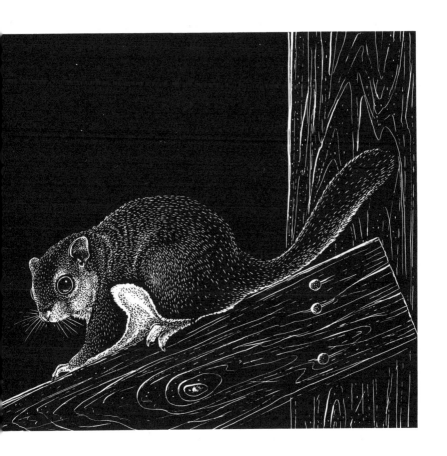

19. *Seeing at Night*

WHERE IS there a civilized man any more who, when the
fading evening twilight grows too dim for him to read his
newspaper, does not say: "Let's switch on the lamp"?
By doing so he misses in the outdoor world the most
exciting hour of the twenty-four—the nighttime changing
of the guard. In the confusion of transition, as day animals
seek sleeping sites in the spreading darkness and night
creatures timidly set out, many an unwary individual becomes a meal for quick-eyed predators that lie in wait.

The skies, patrolled all day by sharp-sighted birds,
become the beat of bats and whippoorwills. In the high

branches, flying squirrels take the place of gray. Deer and skunk glide along woodland paths just vacated by diurnal hopping birds. On lawns and in pastures, the earthworms extend themselves from their burrows for an orgy of feeding and mate finding before dawn sends them slithering below again.

So thoroughly is our own activity geared to use of eyes that we find almost incredible the ability of an eyeless earthworm to respond when illuminated. Yet the worm's sensitivity merely proves that it has retained over much of its body surface a reaction to radiant energy that is a fundamental feature of life. Eyes are actually centers in which this particular sensitivity is exploited through the addition of accessories such as light-concentrating lenses. An eye is an animal's way of getting for its nervous system more meaningful information from the light-sensitive cells.

Our own eyes conceal a dual mechanism. Two unlike populations of light-sensitive cells are integrated into the retina: a hundred million rod cells capable of letting us see at night, and six million and a half cone cells useful to us only under conditions of illumination at least as intense as that from landscape under the full moon. Through skillful use of this dual population we can gain visual information over an intensity range of a billion to one—from shades of lighting visible in puffy white clouds below our airplane, lit by a tropical noonday sun, to a shadowy pathway between the trees in an open woodland illuminated only by the moonless night sky.

In only one area of the human retina are there cone cells but no rod cells. It is the region to which, by day, we automatically bring the image of anything interesting in order to take advantage of the eye's best discrimination for detail. At night, when the cone cells receive too little light to report to the brain, this area is like a little black cloud of which many people are unaware. Country folk, who are used to traveling after dark without the help of artificial lights, learn at an early age how to use their night vision.

Under a moonless starry sky, the surest way to make anything disappear is to look directly at it. With practice, however, a great deal can be learned from the more sensitive rod cells in the peripheral parts of the retina. Particularly from the ring-shaped zone of the retina surrounding the center of our day vision, the human eye provides what we need to detect the coarse patterns of bushes and trees, boulders and other obstacles, or even a striped skunk crossing the path. We stand our best chance to see important features in time if we gaze slightly above or below, or to one side, of each irregularity we notice in the visual scene. As the distinguished French astronomer and physicist Dominique Arago observed more than a century ago, "Pour apercevoir un objet très peu lumineux, il faut ne pas le regarder."

Far more than we show by our habits, we are fitted for activity in the dark. Our eyes are large—actually large, not merely in proportion to our bodies. They are well supplied with highly sensitive rod cells and equipped with an iris which opens promptly in the dark until the pupil at its center is about a third of an inch across.

As long ago as 1773, the English naturalist Gilbert White recognized the importance of eye size when he remarked that "as most nocturnal birds have large eyes and ears, they must have large heads to contain them. Large eyes, I presume, are necessary to collect every ray of light." He was thinking of owls, the pupils of whose big eyes can open wider than those of man. Some kinds of owls pounce directly on a mouse illuminated by only a hundredth as much light as we need to see it. The bird's hearing is so acute, however, that it is difficult to be sure how much the owl depends on vision alone in finding prey at night. It catches camouflaged katydids which make a sound. Even touch may play a part, since the victims include small silent creatures such as worms.

Gilbert White did not realize the degree of enlargement of an owl's eyes. In these exceptional birds, they are so greatly developed that they cannot be turned in their sockets. Instead, they face straight ahead, giving the bird binocular vision but requiring that its entire head be swiveled to change the direction of gaze. Seemingly in consequence, an owl has an extraordinarily flexible neck, capable of turning the head more than a complete circle.

Like the owl, the fox and the cat are well fitted for vision in the dark. They too stalk or watch or cruise with seldom a backward glance, for they fear few enemies. This is rendered easier by the position of their eyes—well forward, with the field of view of each eye overlapping that of the other. They have binocular vision like the owl, and hence double their chance of detecting a potential victim. This likelihood is doubled again in most carnivores by the presence in the eye of a bright mirror. Light entering the eye has one opportunity as it goes in to be absorbed and stimulate vision. If it misses being absorbed, it is reflected by the mirror and sent through the retina again—giving it another chance. In dim illumination this represents a 100 per cent gain for the fox or cat.

The presence of a mirror in a cat's eye accounts for the eyeshine familiar whenever a strong light is shone into the animal's eyes at night. The beam from a flashlamp enters the wide-open pupil and is reflected back again with such intensity that the cat's eyes seem to glow. A similar mirror accounts for the orange eyeshine of bears, the bright yellow of a raccoon, the opalescent green of a bullfrog, and the ruby red of alligators.

Cats of most kinds are like alligators in preferring to prowl for food at night, making full use of their sensitive eyes. But they enjoy basking in the sun as well. To protect the retina from the glare of daylight, each of these animals has a slit pupil. This consists of a pair of curtains which can be drawn apart widely, admitting all light available. By day they can be pulled together until, as in a cat's eye, only a pinhole above and one below represent the slit.

The circular pupil in our own eyes is operated by fine muscles surrounding it in the iris, the colored part of the eye. When the iris opens, the encircling muscles are stretched. But when they contract to close the pupil, they are in their own way. The limit of closure is reached with the pupil still open nearly an eighth of an inch. This is fine for a man who sleeps at night, but would never do for a cat.

It seems to be an engineering impossibility to ask a small eye to see well both by day and by night. Perhaps as a result, bats and many snakes which are abroad in darkness appear to ignore vision altogether. The meadow mouse too, while foraging at night, relies upon scent and touch to guide it to berries and seeds. Vision serves the mouse chiefly in warning it of the approach of an enemy. To help see in all directions simultaneously, the mouse's eye has a greatly enlarged lens that is so nearly spherical as to give the eye periscopic vision. There is no need to focus on anything. Instead, the eye sees poorly from horizon to horizon. It is extremely sensitive to any change in the panoramic field, and warns the mouse to freeze, lest movements or sound betray its position.

How much was Charles Lamb relying upon his eyes after dark when he remarked that he could "read the Lord's prayer in common type, by the help of a candle, without making many mistakes"? No animal can see fine detail in darkness. Fishermen rely upon this difference between day vision and night vision when they use coarser and stronger leaders on their hooked lines after sunset. As the light dims, a fish is unable to distinguish a string against the sky. Comparable changes in human vision became evident to the people of the Near East long before the invention of clocks. Day has come to a Mohammedan minaret when the faithful can distinguish a gray thread from a white, night when neither thread can be seen at all.

The Arabs knew too, from living in close association with their horses, that this animal's prowess in the dark is outstanding—matching the fact that it has the largest eyes of any terrestrial creature. The desert dwellers invented a fable on the subject. According to the story, the lion and the horse got into an argument as to which of them could see better. Finally they called in some neutral judges and asked to be given problems that would settle the dispute. The best the lion could do was to locate a white pearl in a saucer of milk. But the horse picked out a black pearl among coal. The judges decided in favor of the horse.

Does a horse when startled or a lion when hungry see more in the dark than when the pasture is peaceful and the big cat well fed? A man who has engaged in dangerous military operations at night, or has had a ship torpedoed from under him in darkness, has a very different motivation from that of a new recruit or draftee. He is eager to recognize every faint cue his vision can provide, for he realizes that it may well save his life. Yet, despite the most desperate need, no man can hurry his seeing in the dark. To let our rod cells appreciate each scene as fully as they can, we must hold our gaze steady for a few seconds at a time. It is almost as though the eyes were a sponge for light, soaking up impressions from objects in the night.

Actually there is no sharp boundary between the invisible and the visible in darkness. Instead, our threshold for vision becomes a matter of statistics—something a man might bet on. Objects faintly illuminated are seen less often than those reflecting slightly more light, in any reasonable number of opportunities to detect both. This variability stems not from any fluctuations in the eye's readiness to report, but rather from the physical nature of light itself. Radiant energy of all kinds consists of discrete units, emitted or absorbed one at a time, although traveling along a wavelike course. At visual threshold, the number of light units (quanta) absorbed in each tenth of a second is so small that it varies in a statistical way. Whenever this unavoidable variation rises to the level letting adjacent rod cells in a dark-adapted eye absorb two or more units of light in a tenth of a second, enough chemical change occurs to trigger a message to the brain. At its best, our vision is stimulated by almost the least possible energy light can bring.

To be most effective in exciting the human eye in darkness, light must match the physical characteristics of the pale pink pigment in the rod cells. The bleaching of this material serves as the first step in the staircase of chemical reactions leading to the sensation of sight. The pigment (visual purple) absorbs light energy best at one particular wave length in the region of the spectrum we recognize as bluish green when it is intense enough. At threshold for visibility, however, we see no hint of hue. As John Heywood wrote in 1546, "When all candles be out, all cats be gray." A hundred times as much energy at this wavelength is required to stimulate the cone cells, which alone can permit us to distinguish colors.

Over most of the spectrum visible to human eyes, the rod cells are spectacularly more sensitive than the cones. Only in the red does this sensitivity decline until rods and cones need about the same amount of energy to trigger a response. Upon this approximate equality in red, and divergence elsewhere in the spectrum, depends the true magic in red illumination for instruments to be read at night, and in red goggles for people to wear while preparing for night-lookout duty. Only in red light can we use the central part of our visual field for detailed vision in seeing print, maps or indicator dials without disturbing significantly the vulnerable balance of chemical reactions in the rod cells, corresponding to full adaptation for night vision. The forgotten man who selected red as the danger signal for railway semaphores after dark chose more wisely than he knew. If we can locate a red warning lamp at all, we know its color immediately too. No other part of the spectrum reveals its hue to the cone cells at an intensity just sufficient to let our rod cells find it as "a light."

A red warning lamp is very different in the dusk from a hunter's red cap or jacket because the lamp produces its own illumination. The wearing apparel merely reflects what light of day remains. Often the garment's hue, so distinctive in the sun, cannot be seen after sunset; it appears black. This is the reason for the current swing to blaze orange, such as is used on life rafts and many airplanes. Blaze orange is brighter than ordinary pigments because it fluoresces, absorbing energy in other parts of the spectrum and reissuing it as orange. Its color can be seen in illumination too dim for us to distinguish red.

The world shown us by our rod cells at night is very different from that we know from our cone cells by day. Apparently this fact, which anyone can verify easily, was discovered by the Czech physiologist Jan Purkinje one hot summer night more than a century ago. Long before dawn he left his bed and went for a breath of air into the garden. There he entertained himself trying to recognize familiar flowers by what he could see of them in the dark. Purkinje was surprised to find that blue larkspurs, green foliage and some yellow four-o-clocks were easy to locate, whereas he could scarcely make out the orange poppies he had admired by day. The poppies were still open, for he could feel their petals with his fingers.

This observation puzzled Purkinje so much that he

hurried into his laboratory and set up the simple apparatus needed to project on the white wall a complete spectrum the intensity of which he could adjust. When he dimmed it until he could barely make out all of the rainbow colors, the brightest part was definitely in the yellowish green, not far from orange. But when he reduced the intensity still more and let his eyes regain their dark adaptation, not only did the colors fade into neutral grays but the brightest point now lay somewhat toward the end he had previously seen as violet. Holding his pencil at this place, he again increased the intensity until he could once more make out colors. His pencil lay in the bluish green—not in the place he had found brightest when using his retinal cone cells. Here, he realized, lay the explanation for the greater ease with which he could see orange and red flowers by day, and blue ones at night. Night vision centers about the bluish green, with nearly equal sensitivity to blue and green. It permits less awareness of violet and yellow, almost none of orange, and none at all of red. Day vision, on the other hand, is centered about the yellowish green, with only slightly less sensitivity to bluish green and orange, and less—but still useful—response for blue and red. Violet and deep red have to be intense to be noticed.

Animals of the night see no more color than Purkinje did in his garden. Moreover, they rarely possess many cone cells in their eyes. Consequently they are red-blind as well as color-blind. Knowing this, we tried to take advantage of our pet flying squirrel. Over her cage we hung a deep red lamp, and waited until she emerged for her nightly gadabout. All other house lights were off, and the curtains drawn. The squirrel had nothing to see by. If diffused illumination from other rooms had been coming through the door, our pet would have noticed us at once and leaped to our clothing or to an outstretched hand. She was by all odds the gentlest little animal we had ever known. Yet, with only red light and unable to use her eyes, she jumped back in alarm when we touched her and bit us in self-defense.

In its outdoor haunts a flying squirrel has faint illumination on the darkest night—from the sky, the stars or perhaps the moon. Its long whiskers and its senses of scent and taste must be useful at close range. Its hearing may be good. But only eyes will give a leaping animal the accurate information it needs high above the ground, or let a squirrel reach a distant tree trunk in one airy glide. Despite their strictly nocturnal habits, flying squirrels are just as eye-minded as we are.

At night an owl's large eyes give it a little better vision at its best than ours. Yet the owl too is red-blind. At Oxford University Botanic Garden, Dr. H. N. Southern benefited from this by hanging a deep red lamp just above the nest hole where a pair of tawny owls was raising a family. Night after night he sat comfortably in his chair, with field glasses trained on the doorway, and used his own red vision to keep count of the prey the parent owls brought their young. So far as the owls were concerned, the night had not been changed. But Southern was able to discover an unsuspected item in owl menus: earthworms! Subsequently, ornithologists all over the world verified that night crawlers are indeed a favorite food of owls.

Fishermen, who hunt night crawlers at the same hours as owls do, know that the worms are insensitive to red light. Using a flashlamp shielded with a red filter, the angler can approach within snatching distance of worms extended at night from their burrows in the lawn. Any other color of light would affect the microscope sense organs in the earthworm's skin. Actually, these creatures have two separate sets of sense cells warning them in relation to light. One set, most sensitive to blue, sends the worm back into its tunnel at the first brightening of dawn. The other set is useful when the worm remains extended in faint light. Any shadow, decreasing this illumination, causes the worm to contract. For this, the earthworm's sensitivity is greatest in the yellow. Maybe it protects the crawler from owls on moonlight nights.

Recently, when a pair of monkeylike bush babies from Africa was received at the Bronx Zoo, a new approach to display was tried. The officials arranged a special cage in the basement of the lion house, where artificial light was needed even in the daytime. Then, at ten o'clock in the morning, a switch automatically turned off the white lights that had been shining in the cage all night, leaving only a fifteen-watt red lamp these animals could not see. Within a few minutes, both bush babies were scampering about the cage, making prodigious leaps and displaying the twelve-inch bushy tails on their eight-inch bodies. Immediately the idea of a nocturnal house was born—one in which bush babies, flying squirrels and owls could all be watched under red illumination in an artificial night during the middle of man's day.

Now we want to go back to some places where we blundered into interesting animals at night, seeing them only momentarily in the beam of our white flashlamp. Suppose, instead, we had had powerful red lights that night on the Natal coast, when we accompanied a game warden looking for poachers. How many African bush babies would we have seen active, instead of just two huddled in terror where our bright flashlight beams caught them at the top of a slender stump? Their shrill, babylike cries came from all around us. And what about Panama, where we glimpsed an old honeybear (kinkajou) and two quarter-ton tapirs on a trail? How much more would we have seen in red lighting that did not disturb them? Perhaps we wouldn't have to go so far to use a ruby lamp. Can a whippoorwill see red light?

We can play tricks at night on many a nocturnal creature. But our own eyes deceive us too, even with objects that are bright enough to see easily. Who has not remarked how big the full moon appears when first it rises, perhaps orange as a pumpkin, over the black filigree of trees along the horizon? Yet, when the same moon is more nearly overhead five or six hours later, it seems to have shrunk. If we see it setting after dawn, we get less of this illusion of greater size. Actually, the moon at the horizon is slightly farther away from our eyes than when it is high in the sky. If anything, it should appear smaller!

Part of the moon illusion, at least, arises from our lack of experience in judging the size of objects overhead. Part may come from failure to realize how far away the satellite is, beyond the horizon, as we try to apply to it the same kind of judgment through which we recognize an apple as being "apple-sized" whether it is in the hand or twenty

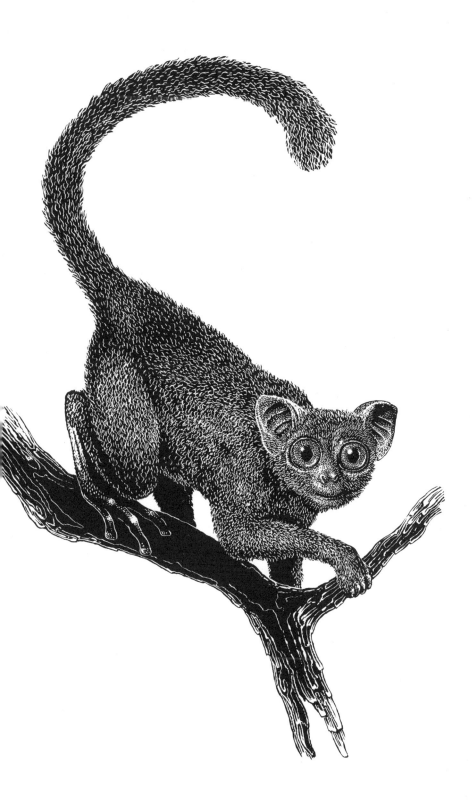

feet away. As we grow older, our misjudgment of the moon decreases but never disappears. If asked to choose in darkness an illuminated disk among several of different sizes at eye level, to match an illuminated disk at the same distance overhead, we invariably select a smaller one than we should—usually about a sixth less in diameter than the one above us.

Night alters the responses of many other animals to light, in ways we cannot yet explain. Why should a moth, which remains inactive in a uniformly illuminated room, take to its wings by the light of a single candle and fly a spiral course ending in the flame? Why do small crustaceans and many kinds of fishes cluster around a lamp dangled from a boat to a depth of a few feet below the water surface? If an area the size of a swimming pool is uniformly illuminated, virtually none of these aquatic denizens will come into sight.

That we see no significant difference between a large illuminated area and a small brilliant spot of light from an underwater lamp or a candle flame is no proof that crustaceans and insects respond in a comparable way. Almost certainly they do not, for the simple reason that they have compound eyes. A crustacean or an insect is somewhat like a nearsighted human being, unable to see the moon distinctly. For the compound eye, the half degree subtended by the full moon (or the sun) may not fill the visual field of any light-sensitive unit. The brilliance produced by moon or sun on sea or land may stimulate the animal, while the celestial bodies themselves are overlooked completely.

This relationship between size of object and its interest for an animal with compound eyes is apparent with a butterfly in a dark room with black walls. If a bare electric bulb is turned on, the butterfly will flit toward it. Even if the insect's wings are clipped together to prevent flight, the butterfly will creep in the direction of the bulb. But if a sheet of white paper is held close to the insect on the side opposite the bulb, the butterfly will turn around and walk toward the paper. The bulb is far brighter, but the paper it illuminates has a larger area that stimulates more units of the compound eye. This is the creature's guide, and the basis for many of the paradoxes that hinder us from seeing eye-to-eye with three-quarters of the animal kingdom.

A seemingly comparable enigma offers a real hazard for men piloting blacked-out aircraft on secret night missions. Unless they have an illuminated instrument panel or some other means for keeping a constant plane of reference (and perhaps distraction), they may concentrate upon a bright star or the exhaust glow of an accompanying airplane long enough so that the isolated spot of light appears to start wandering on its own. A man seated firmly in an armchair, staring at a single star-sized spot of light in an otherwise black room, can encounter the same sensation. What causes this "autokinetic" phenomenon that has induced competent night-fighter pilots to make needless flight adjustments, ending in crashes or collisions? What does darkness do to the human mind and eye?

In the twinkling of a faint star and the flashing of a firefly's beacon lay one practical solution, letting aviation physiologists get around this problem. Wingtip lamps on aircraft now wink and break the spell. Instrument panels are lit with red lamps which do not destroy the pilot's dark adaptation, yet let him see beyond the reference frame of his cockpit. Yet vision by night still offers plenty of other scientific challenges.

To evaluate our versatile, although limited, visual sense, we can compare our eyes with those of other animals. Suppose that we could "swap even." With what other animal would we be willing to trade eyes? Perhaps the horse—able to see well both by day and night—or the lion, or the seal, or the owl? We would have to give up color vision if we exchanged with any of these, and would no longer be able to read the fine print at the bottom of a contract. Possibly with the ostrich, or the eagle, or the octopus? They all have color vision, but cannot see well after dark. If we insist on retaining all of our present advantages—night vision, color vision and fine resolution by day—about the only candidate for a swap would be the gorilla. Would we be any better off?

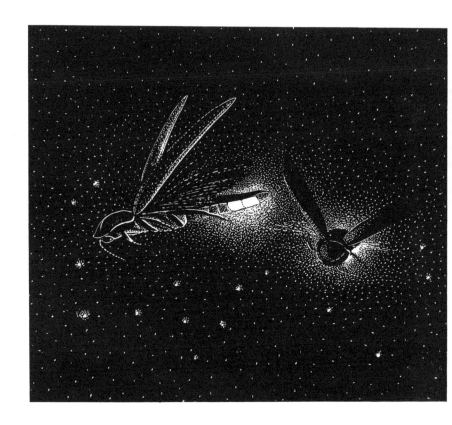

20. *Animals with Flashlamps*

FOR GETTING about at night, man can rely upon his sensitive eyes or dispel the darkness by making light. Almost all of his fellow creatures, however, spend half their lives in darkness. Eyes modified toward extreme sensitivity and luminescent organs are common only in the depths of the sea, where we rarely meet them. Is this why we regard with wonder the fireflies we see in the fields on a summer night?

From the very beginning, the common firefly *Lampyris* glows softly in the dark. Its freshly laid eggs shine with an inner light. What possible advantage could this confer? Or for the glowworm to have little luminous spots on its back? Even Shakespeare wondered about its "uneffectual fire." Only when the glowworm transforms into an adult firefly do the winkable tail lights become part of a communication system, suggesting the blinker beacons on ships in darkness. The female firefly perched on a leaf tip can summon a passing mate by flashing at the correct time interval after he has broadcast a luminous message. With his extra-large eyes, he sees her signal. He turns in his flight, and comes in for a landing beside her.

Occasionally the flash from a leaf tip invites the flying male to a female that is not of his own kind. She has winked too soon or too late, and in this way trespassed on the communication band of another species. Usually the ardent male pays for her mistake with his life, for a firefly that cannot become a suitor is merely a meal for her.

Perhaps the firefly males in Burma and adjacent parts of the Far East have evolved a more foolproof system. Night after night, on the leaf tips of jungle trees, they flash in unison. The whole forest pulsates as though from the blinking of a Broadway signboard, and it is up to the females to approach if they are willing, sexually acceptable and physically fit. Their night vision is as important as that of the flashing suitors. Indeed, they have equally large eyes.

For animals abroad in darkness to find one another at mating season by vision and flashing lights seems so logical that we must marvel at its rarity. Except for the fireflies on land, the chief practitioners of this signal system are sea creatures, such as the fireworms which swarm at night in waters off Bermuda. Female fireworms propel themselves on an upward-slanting course from the coral reefs among which they reached maturity. As they rise, loaded with ripe eggs, they light up like passenger trains ascending a long grade through dark mountains. Smaller males cavort like comets, writing little streaks and dashes of luminescence just below the surface until they meet a mate. Then comes one matching flare of light, and both parents fade into the black waters while the fertilized eggs of a new generation cascade gently toward the bottom.

Most luminescent creatures that produce light under predictable circumstances do so as though each sudden flash were a warning, like the STOP signal at the back of an automobile. The parchment worm, snug in its U-shaped burrow near low-tide mark, responds in this way to the jarring of human footsteps along the muddy beach at night. The rock-boring clam *Pholas* reacts to disturbance with a similar blaze of light. Even the delicate comb jellies and pulsing jellyfishes may luminesce when swirled by the near-hit of an oar or a boat. Several kinds of small crustaceans in surface waters of the ocean, and some squids at greater depth, show their alarm by flooding out a cloud of luminescent particles while they themselves swim off in darkness.

Man looks for a reason in all of these displays. He would like to see that enemies veer off when confronted by the unexpected light. Yet few observations support this notion. In one instance after another, luminescence of individual animals seems unrelated to vision in any way that would have survival value. The rock-boring clam and the parchment worm appear to gain no more from their light production than the English barn owl that flies about like a luminous ghost because its feathers are still dusted with foxfire—the light-producing fungus growing in the damp tree hole the owl regards as home.

Those people who risk the sharks for a swim in coastal seas at the dark of the moon in summer usually know how the water can scintillate with tiny points of light, each brief spark marking the irritation of a single *Noctiluca* cell measuring from a hundredth to a tenth of an inch across. The quietest lapping of wavelets along the shore is enough to churn *Noctiluca* into action. Along the California coast under the darkest sky, we have watched entranced while whole breakers raced toward us, glowing from myriads of similar luminescent creatures, as though some master showman had installed fluorescent lighting in the water. Or, above the blackness of Puerto Rico's Phosphorescent Bay, our eyes have followed the progress of fishes dashing from our launch, each trailing a plume of luminescence as though it were a rocket. On a small scale we too were enjoying the "wonderful and most beautiful spectacle" Charles Darwin described when the historic H.M.S. *Beagle* "drove before her bows two billows of liquid phosphorus, and in her wake she was followed by a milky train."

What does luminescence mean to a *Noctiluca?* These seemingly simple creatures will not perform their magic until they have had a chance to adjust to darkness. They are sensitive to daylight, just as we are. But so far chemists have learned the full sequence of reactions for neither the processes by which living things produce light nor those responsible for vision. Both chemical staircases remain secrets hidden in the protoplasm of a remarkable variety of plants and animals. Luminescence, especially, is found as haphazardly as though a handful of sand had been cast over the complete roster of life. "Where each grain of sand strikes, a luminous species appears." So concluded the most eminent student of animal light—the late E. Newton Harvey.

If the meaning of warning flashes is not that individual animals are driven away by a surprising light, perhaps luminescence still has a mass significance. We ourselves gain no picture from the scintillation of radioactive materials as seen through a microscope. Yet a whole area, yielding countless flashes to the unaided eye, becomes luminous enough for us to estimate its shape and distance away. Should we not look into the blackness of the sea, where luminescence is commoner than anywhere else, for additional clues that might give us the answer?

Fishermen and other sailors who habitually spend the night over ocean waters are well aware that the sea shows bright "pools" in darkness. Charles Darwin hazarded the guess that these areas marked concentrations of decay, comparable to those on land where bacteria and fungi glow feebly. Sardine fishermen know better. At night, the lookout in the crow's nest on the mast of a sardine fishing boat will watch for bright pools, ready to guide the vessel to their vicinity. Then, cautiously, the fishermen in dinghies will encircle the luminous area with a net and purse together its bottom, capturing a whole school of fishes intent on raiding the small rice-sized crustaceans that browse near the surface in darkness. The men care nothing for the multitude of small creatures which slip through the mesh, still flashing their distress signals. What good does all this luminescence do when no fishermen are there to take away the hungry fishes?

Most of the small crustaceans upon which the fishes feed seem repelled by daylight. Long before the sun shows at the eastern horizon, the crustaceans are swimming downward, following the edge of twilight into depths as great as twelve hundred feet. By noon all will have reached their farthest point. Sunset finds them rushing up again, to feast on microscopic plants drifting in waters lit by each day's sun. A full moon holds them below a hundred feet or so, whereas a dark night lets incredible numbers reach the surface. When a flying fish that has been feeding on these crustaceans is opened quickly, its stomach is found to be packed with a mass of still-luminous bodies.

The daily vertical migrations of the small crustaceans are matched by upward and downward movements of two-inch fishes and an assortment of prawnlike crustaceans, all of which prey on the small crustaceans. These fishes and prawnlike crustaceans can be caught by day in fine-mesh nets towed in the upper zones of the bathic depths to which no daylight has ever penetrated. From his many hauls with nets at these levels, Dr. William Beebe computed that two-thirds of the kinds of fishes and 965 in each thousand individuals swimming there carry lights, displaying them more or less constantly. Many of these denizens are slender black lanternfishes and special light-bearing crustaceans known to whalers as "krill"—a major food of whalebone whales.

Most of the light bearers in the midwater depths look upward as well as to all sides, but shine their own lights downward. Probably the distinctive pattern of bright spots low on each individual's body enables neighbors of the same kind to recognize it in the darkness. Yet the direction the light-producing organs face may offer an important clue.

The British oceanographer Dr. John S. Colman suspects that all of these luminescent creatures are intercommunicating in a social way. To him the key lies in the habits of the grain-sized crustaceans that migrate vertically on a schedule laid out by an internal clock, subject only to the repelling effect of light. As these dancing hordes, which have been waiting on the fringe of twilight in the depths, start upward in late afternoon, the lanternfishes and krill crustaceans feeding on them follow after. Until that moment, the topmost level of lanternfishes and krill has been providing a general illumination for those lower down, like a softly-lit ceiling deep in the underwater world. As the ceiling rises, due to the upward movement of the lanternfishes and krill crustaceans, the light from these creatures would be reduced for all below them. As the ceiling illumination dims, the lower lanternfishes and krill no doubt move upward too, changing the light below their level in turn. The combination of upward vision and downward light production could unify the upward migration in this way, without any individual luminescent organs having a separate significance.

In a similar way, the massed scintillations of small creatures near the surface, while being raided by carnivorous fishes, may well serve as a warning that keeps deeper migrants from rising higher. It would almost certainly affect the same light-sensitive organs as permit response to a full moon.

In seeking a significance for separate flashes or for the light-producing organs of individual crustaceans and fishes are we not showing a peculiarly human tendency? We bias our interest consistently toward the welfare of the solitary animal, rather than think of it as merely part of a large population. Among ourselves, this is natural enough, because of our long life and comparatively low reproductive rate. What each human being does is important. But can the individual be so meaningful in underwater populations reproducing prodigiously, generation following generation only a few weeks apart? Except on a statistical basis, how does a flashed warning or the general illumination from a row of light-producing spots affect the welfare of the species? Survival or extinction is statistical, the outcome of evolutionary pressures on animals. Man escapes this mass fate to the degree that he controls his own environment and directs his individual destiny.

Only recently has man had the specialized equipment with which to explore the deep sea, lowering instruments among the luminescent animals and measuring their light output. These devices show that the general illumination would have to be increased 160-fold to stimulate our eyes at their most sensitive, and that this light in the depths has a spectrum richest in the greenish blue.

Delicate as these instruments are, they do not tell what actually is happening in the black water. They would be equally inadequate in a huge cavern through which a hundred fireflies flit, winking their tail lamps, while upon the floor a thousand little birthday candles flicker, each well separated from the next. In both situations, the scene would seem bright to our eyes, entranced by all the points of light. Our eyes and brain can ignore the blackness between the luminous areas, whereas the meter mechanism adds up all the dark and light, then indicates the average— barely above zero on the most sensitive scale. In the deep sea the instruments fail to show that individual flashes from luminescent creatures are well into our visual range, or that they come from microscopic bacteria and luminous protists, from dark red abyssal jellyfishes, from the multi-colored spots on fishes and crustaceans, and from the glowing coral heads, sea whips, sea fans, sea plumes, serpent stars and other fascinating animals upon the bottom.

We can wonder whether fishes, squids and crustaceans in the deep sea are able to utilize the general illumination— this faint abyssal equivalent of the sky glow at night over our cities. Or do predators in the luminous haze detect prey only as individuals when each comes within snapping distance? Fishes in the abysses do have a different visual pigment from ours. It is golden in color, instead of a pale pinkish purple, and absorbs energy most readily in the greenish blue. In this way it matches almost perfectly the light available from the luminescent animals.

Deep-sea fishes include several kinds that have eyes larger in proportion to body size than is to be found in any other animals with backbones. The diameter of a black-smelt's eye is often more than half the length of its head. In other abyssal fishes, a huge spherical lens is confined in an eye of more manageable size only because the eyeball is cylindrical, and hence shaped like a telescope. A large lens, whether in eye or telescope, can capture a generous sample from any light available, and concentrate it. By lacking an iris, moreover, these deep-sea eyes gain in light-admitting power until their optical systems become equivalent to that of the fastest camera lenses (f/1.0). This is a little better than a cat's eye at its widest aperture, and three times as good as ours when our pupils are fully open (f/3.0).

Almost all of these abyssal fishes gain in other ways we cannot match. Merely by being immersed in water, rather than exposed to air, they are exempt from losing about a twentieth of the light energy reaching the eye. This much is reflected by the tear-wet surface of a human eye or a cat's eye in air, without ever entering the optical system. Then too, a fish's eye can have a more transparent lens, for it needs none of the yellow color we use in filtering out harmful ultraviolet radiations from sunlight. In deep-sea fishes, these advantages are combined with a mirror backing to the light-sensitive cells, adding still further to the likelihood of seeing in faint illumination.

A single successful trawling through the midwater depths can bring to the surface enough astonishing fishes to convince almost anyone how different life must be in the eternal night below. Every conceivable modification of eyes seems to be used by some deep-sea fish. This certainly was our conclusion as we examined one netful hauled freshly from four-fifths of a mile below the surface of the Pacific Ocean, barely out of sight of San Diego, California. It held twenty-two different kinds of fishes, most of them light-bearing bristlemouths. The smaller ones had shapes and names utterly unfamiliar to surface fishermen: bigscales, smoothtongues, slickheads, fangtooths, dragonfishes, hatchetfishes and lampfishes. Only five specimens reached six inches in length: two snipe eels, a witch eel, a blacksmelt and a blackdragon.

The slender six-inch blackdragon recalled for us the discovery Dr. William Beebe made in Bermudan waters with a similar deep-sea denizen from the Atlantic. Blackdragons go through a metamorphosis so elaborate that no one suspected the different stages to be related until every step was laid out in a single tray of specimens. Young blackdragons hatch far up toward the surface, where they have opportunities to feed on tiny crustaceans. The blackdragon larvae are white thread-thin creatures from the sides of whose head extend two incredibly long slender

stalks each ending in a knoblike eye. By the time the larva
has grown from five-eighths of an inch to an inch and a
half, the eyestalks have shrunk to barely more than the
length of the head—instead of half the length of the body.
The firm rod that supported each long stalk folds up neatly
in the eye socket of the skull, and soon the growing eye
comes to rest on top as though it had never been carried
on an outrigger. During these transformations, the blackdragon has been sinking deeper, catching larger prey, and
becoming better able to use faint illumination. We have
no difficulty guessing that blackdragon eggs, when released in the dark depths, are ballasted to match the
density of the sea water high above the adult fishes. But
why the larval eyes should go through such drastic changes
remains as much a mystery as ever.

The world of the deep sea extends upward to within less
than half a mile of man's shipping lanes. Yet it remains the
least understood part of all the regions where life can
exist. While the overlying ocean water absorbs the daylight and keeps the depths blacker than any night, it seems
also to alter the logic of sensory adaptations. Does luminescence introduce some limitation we have not appreciated, perhaps one linked to the efficient chemistry that
releases energy almost completely in the form of light, with
scarcely any accompanying heat? Here in the depths we
find fishes, squids and crustaceans with fine luminous
organs. They are all meat-eating animals—professional
opportunists preying on each other or scavenging for
corpses sinking from above. Their mouths and stomachs
are often capable of astonishing extension, letting them
swallow bodies larger in diameter than their own. Days
or weeks must pass between meals in the cold dense water.
Why then, with so great a need for food and so wide a
variety of light-producing organs, have the abyssal hunters
developed no true searchlights? After man mastered fire,
how long did it take him to cup a pale hand behind a
burning twig and use the feeble light while hunting for
something in the dark? Where are the luminescent equivalents of striking a match or pointing a flashlamp?

It is true that many of the luminous spots animals carry
are as dim as the radium-coated markings on a wristwatch

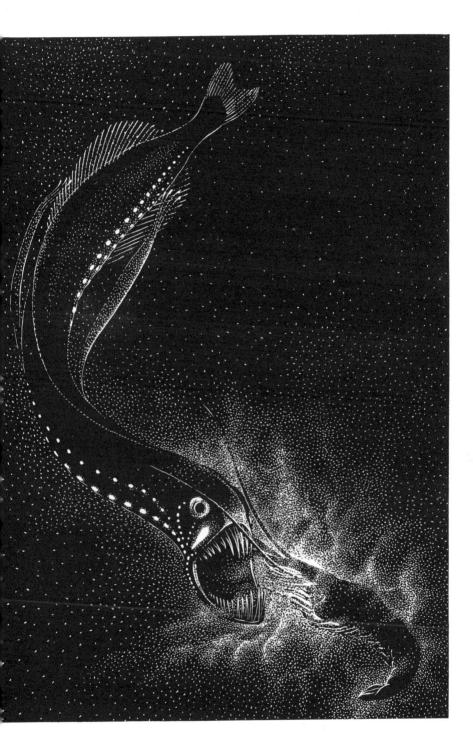

dial. They could never serve as lanterns, no matter where they were located on the body. To prove that other luminescent organs are adequately powerful, however, we need only set one of the common fireflies on a page of newsprint in a dark room. At each flash the words become visible all around the insect, except near its head. Yet a firefly's beacon is a fairly simple one, with no lens to concentrate the energy into a narrow beam. Whenever the insect combines two complex chemical compounds within special cells, light is emitted. It shines through transparent windows in the lower body wall, its intensity increased somewhat by a mirrorlike layer covering the top of the luminescent organ.

Crustaceans and fishes in the sea have far more refined luminous areas. Most of them are mirror-backed. Many are covered by a clear lens. A few might even suggest a miner's lamp, illuminating objects in the visual field, except for the fact that luminescent organs near the eyes appear either to be feeble or to shine in directions toward which the eye is blind. Some of the prawnlike crustaceans of the deep sea wear luminous areas on their stalked eyes in such a way that any movement of the stalk and eye must be matched by a corresponding shift in the direction toward which the light shines. None of them, however, is known to use its luminescent organs as spotlights with which to find prey or to see it just before attacking it.

Scientists examining the eyes of deep-sea creatures have been astonished to find a few instances in which the light-emitting organ seems to shine into the eye itself. Could vision profit from a "pilot light" like those on appliances burning natural gas? Most sense organs can respond to stimuli each of which is inadequate alone, providing they "pile up" one after another in a brief time. Just as great glaciers can accumulate from repeated residues of unmelted snow, the nervous system can accumulate a sensation. If an abyssal animal flashes an imperceptible light into its own eye just before some faintly illuminated prey passes near, it might improve its own chance of getting food.

Despite the billions of fireflies collected by children and ground up by chemists seeking to learn more about the light-producing compounds, the whole action of animal luminescence remains as tantalizing and elusive as a will-o'-the-wisp. It is tempting to conclude that the few creatures using luminous organs in mate-finding and social interplay are exceptional, that light-production otherwise is no more meaningful than in a bacterium or a fungus plant. Instead, we keep searching for something else that goes with luminescence, something that will provide a satisfying explanation for the light we see.

VII

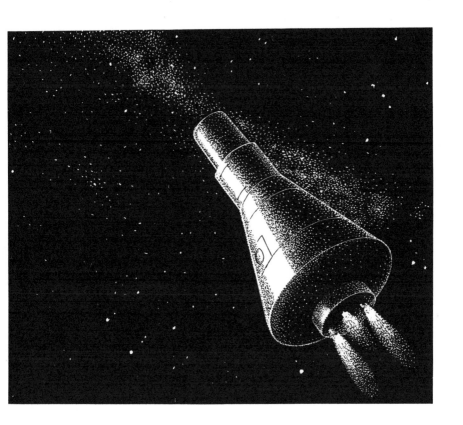

21. *Survival*

NEITHER MAN nor animal seems to exploit fully the available ways for achieving advantages over competitors. Particularly is this true in the degree to which senses are used. Each kind of creature reacts to only a small sample from among the wealth of information reaching its nervous system. It ignores the remaining multitude of changes in its environment.

We often recognize this self-imposed limitation among familiar animals, and overlook it in our own behavior. How differently each of us examines the scene before us! Confronted with a bit of rolling Pennsylvania farmland, a farmer sees acres of specific crops and judges the way they grow. A naturalist thinks of the identifiable plants and animals living there, and of the unstable web of food relationships among them. An artist delights in the pastel pattern from foreground to sky. A geologist finds, instead, an erosion pattern from which he can mentally reconstruct the past history of the land and predict its natural future. A builder appraises the contours, considering how an army of machines might lay out streets of homes within commuting distance of the nearest city.

Where is the common denominator in all of these human responses to identical stimulation of visual sense? How could the great German philosopher Nietzsche hold that "From the senses come all trustworthiness, all good conscience, and all evidence of truth"? Must we conclude that trustworthiness, conscience and truth have as many forms as there are people in the world? No single concept of our universe can be completely convincing to all of mankind, because each of us lives in a private world. We judge every sensory impression in a peculiarly personal way, based upon our previous experiences. No two individuals have the same experiences, even when they are brought up in one household. Nor are any two people, unless they are identical twins, exactly alike in refinements of sensory perception. Rarely are we aware how these personal differences circumscribe our views.

In trying to assess the sensory world of any other animal, we encounter still greater differences. We may be fooled into feeling kinship when we see a mother hen hurrying to rescue from a thin-walled cloth cage a chick she can hear peeping but not see. Our error in attributing human reactions to the hen becomes apparent when the same bird ignores her chick after we put it in a glass enclosure with sound-proof walls. The chick can see her and she must see the chick, for she will try to get through the glass if grain is sprinkled at the chick's feet. But her reactions then are solely to the food—something that appeals to her visual centers. Hearing is the only avenue to her protective instinct.

Sometimes it is hard to accept a simple system of communication as it stands. It must, we feel sure, have refinements of which we are still unaware. Often we forget how unusual are the situations in which we place an animal while studying it, and how little the limitations we find mean for it under free conditions.

At other times we take for granted a complex natural behavior without wondering how it operates. Which bird, for example, leads a flock of pigeons on the wing? How do these fliers co-ordinate their fast three-dimensional ballets? Certainly their progress is never the disorganized fluttering of a shower of leaves from a tree in autumn. Pigeons scrupulously avoid collisions, even when some members in a flock seemingly ignore the rest while engaging in aerial acrobatics—tumbling and somersaulting backward, as though with joyous abandon or reveling in their freedom. But is it joy? Can a sense of freedom be bred for? Pigeon breeders, who developed the tumbler strain, make no such claim. Perhaps a tumbler pigeon tumbles because of some recurrent defect in its flight co-ordination.

Under ordinary circumstances, each wild animal has a repertoire of reactions to sensory cues that is adequate for normal needs as they arise. Often the creature manages emergency situations, as though understanding them. Yet so simple are the signs to which its senses are attuned that variations we would take in stride trigger only the wrong response.

Despite these limitations, the sensory world of each kind of animal must be adequate for its survival. Somehow its nervous system combines an unconscious awareness of all the processes inside the body, and modifies responses to the outside world according to the state of its various inner hungers. Within a large brain, such as our own, memories of past experiences enter the nervous circuits and still further adjust the actions we take.

Size alone, of course, is no measure. A bat which migrates year after year between Newfoundland and Georgia with no known reliance upon visual cues has a brain scarcely larger than the eraser on a lead pencil. The nervous system of a monarch butterfly could be balanced by a millet seed. The control centers of a fruit fly would scarcely cover the period at the end of this sentence. Yet these creatures are all capable of complicated actions. They have survived just as long and just as well as we. Their adaptability, moreover, seems limitless. Every time a man builds a better mousetrap, the surviving mice build better mice.

We like to believe that human survival has depended upon our conscious appraisal of the world we live in, and upon our ability to modify that world in our immediate vicinity. The clothes we wear, the homes we live in, the forests and hills we level are all a measure of our control over our environment. Today we pride ourselves on the degree to which gadgets and machines are taking over routines in life, from the manufacture of articles to the supervision of sleeping children. Increasingly we relegate man to the role of devising more efficient ways to use machines, or to meeting emergencies when they arise. We try to plan in such detail that emergencies become rare.

Our way of life is changing so rapidly through applications of scientific principles to technological problems that many of the world's most distinguished thinkers are perplexed to see where the changes are leading us. Britain's Sir Charles (C. P.) Snow claims the present to be a Scientific Revolution, ranking with the Industrial Revolution which began two centuries ago. Dr. René Dubos at the Rockefeller Institute for Medical Research wonders whether some of the diseases now encountered in civilized countries are symptoms of the jet age. Could they arise from loss of regularity—in time, light, temperature and geographical location—from the environment in which man evolved? We turn night into day at the flick of a switch, or let an automatic mechanism do it for us. If we remain in one place, we fix the temperature and humidity indoors to provide the weather of springtime all year long. When we travel, we may speed up the clock or set it back half a day in a few hours on a jet airplane going east or west. And we shift our geographical location so rapidly that we have no time to become aware of one environment before we are in an utterly different one.

For the first time in history, travelers have experienced minute after minute of complete weightlessness—with gravitational force nullified. Men and scientific instruments have traveled beyond the earth's atmosphere, beyond the blanket of air that protects us from all radiations from the universe save only the light, radio and cosmic rays to which it is transparent. With huge radio telescopes, men have located invisible sources of electric messages from space. With smoothly revolving turntables, the rotation of the planet itself has effectively ceased for hamsters and other small animals under observation at the South Pole; these creatures were turned counterclockwise at exactly the same speed the earth rotated in the opposite direction, making the sun stand still for them in a way that Joshua might have envied.

We replace the old-time environment with a new kind, and gamble our survival upon the proper working of machines. We have machines that make machines, and computers that calculate the designs for new machines. If we rely upon computers and gadgets in making our decisions, where does the responsibility lie for any mistake? Or will man retain his accountability because he instructs the machine, and perhaps must repair it whenever it breaks down? It might be possible to build a device that would repair itself. How complex must a machine be to show versatility equal to that of a human being? Machine diagnosis of human ills has already been proposed to supplement or replace the physician.

Before we become used to replacing human senses with machines, we should be sure that the change is in our best interests. Already many people are too busy with their own affairs to be alert to the quiet, elementary voices of the world. We cannot set man upon a shelf, doing nothing and without stimulation of any kind until an emergency arises—not if we expect him to stay sane and cope with the emergency. Volunteers who were convinced they needed a vacation from the pressures of modern life found quickly that they could tolerate only a few hours of being really cut off from the world. Under the direction of Dr. John Rader Platt, professor of physics at the University of Chicago, these men were floated in a tank of warm water, their hands covered by gloves that prevented each finger from touching anything else, their ears subjected to only a low steady hum, their eyes covered with translucent material transmitting a constant dim glow of neutral light. They received food whenever they asked for it. But without stimulation they could not concentrate. Man's need for novelty is as real as his need for air, water, food and safety. Although we do not understand the marvelous mechanism of the mind, it is abundantly clear today that a person is himself only in relation to the sensory encouragement of his normal environment.

For this reason, the planners of space flights give careful thought to work for astronauts to do while in transit. On a seven-day simulated trip to the moon and back, an airman at Randolph Air Force Base in Texas was asked to match his activities to a fourteen-hour cycle: four and a half hours for sleep, half an hour for breakfast and personal hygiene, four hours of work, half an hour for lunch, four hours more of work, and a half hour for supper before sleeping again. Perhaps we can see a change in this program—a speeding up of modern life. More than twenty years ago in Mammoth Cave, Kentucky, Dr. Nathaniel Kleitman and a student tried to adapt themselves to an artificial day. But instead of making it shorter than twenty-four hours, they chose to follow a twenty-eight-hour cycle. Within seven days the student's body temperature was rising and falling in time with the new schedule, instead of the customary one following a solar clock. Dr. Kleitman, however, was finding that forty-three years of living on a twenty-four-hours-a-day schedule made the habit hard to break.

Probably we should feel encouraged that America's first man into space had useful tasks to perform en route. They could have been important to his own survival, and were not just busy work while he passively rode the rocket. Nor was his attention limited to dials and flashing lights within the capsule. As soon as his craft got beyond the atmosphere, he extended a periscope and exclaimed at his view of the receding earth: "What a beautiful sight!" Even on a short trip, during which taste and olfactory centers had no challenges, the sense of wonder evoked an emotional reaction from highly trained Commander Alan B. Shepard, Jr.

For pioneer ventures such as this, we enlist the best minds and the fittest bodies that can be found. Survival and success depend upon the genius of the planners and the balanced co-ordination of the participant. But what is genius? John Ruskin identified it as "a superior power of seeing." William James regarded it as an unusual ability to perceive analogies, an extreme sensitivity to resemblances that enables a person to use insight in new situations. Genius lets a man cope with sudden change as rapidly as his senses advise him that it is taking place.

Change in cultural directions, rather than in physical ones, has been the mode of progress in human evolution. Admittedly we live longer than our ancestors. We grow taller, have bigger feet and tend to lose our "wisdom teeth" because of changes in environment and habits, such as diet. But will our sense organs, like our wisdom teeth, atrophy if we use them less and less in cultured communities? We've never solved the riddle as to whether blind cave animals lost their eyes from lack of use after generations in the dark, or are the descendants from blind creatures that blundered into caves and survived only in complete darkness. Are we engineering adventures out of life? Adventures are what we need our senses for. Our savage ancestors depended on their senses every hour of every day.

Today, as never before, we recognize our sensory limitations, although we have no way to tell if they have narrowed in recent centuries. We hear a panther's scream, but not the echoing staccato chirps of hunting bats. We admire the red rose, but cannot detect the ultraviolet reflections which alone can attract to it a red-blind honeybee. Our skin tells us nothing of the delicate electrical sensing system of a lamprey, although we respond to the strong discharges from rays and fishes able to stun small creatures for food. We can appreciate the radiant glow of a hot stove, but not the faint radiations with which a pit viper finds prey in darkness.

Momentarily we may feel humbled by the discovery of sensory abilities in other animals exceeding our own. But we regain our confidence when we realize that no other animal excels us in the richness of its sensory world. No other animal has reached out to borrow senses, as we have. Our curiosity and our desire to control our environment for human benefit have led to the invention of instruments with which we probe in many new directions. Today's world is a fresh environment for mankind. By extending our senses, we have altered the frontiers for our own survival.

One limitation seems likely to remain a boundary we cannot completely bypass. Britain's great neurophysiologist Sir Charles Sherrington recognized it. He pointed out that man's body has genetic continuity with all predecessors throughout the immensity of geological time, whereas man's brain must start at the beginning, with each new individual learning to interpret the environment. The body can evolve, whereas the mind can grasp its surroundings better with each succeeding generation only to the extent that it is ready to benefit from the sensory experiences of predecessors and contemporaries. Our civilization serves to pass this heritage to each ready mind.

A whole scale of readiness to gain from the experiences of others can be discerned, from the person who insists that only his own senses can be relied upon to the scholar who quotes from published statements rather than credit his own eyes and ears. Thoreau tended toward the one extreme and Pliny, the Roman encyclopedist, toward the opposite. Does not the radical nationalist ardently wish to start from scratch, gambling his own survival upon being able to ignore the wisdom accumulated from the past? Is not the world of his forefathers "good enough" for the true conservative? But is man not being equally provincial, inviting history to repeat itself, if he relies upon human experience alone in seeking to progress? In the bodies and ways of life of the animals with which we share the earth are countless features that could serve as stimulating hints from which a scientific mind might leap ahead, improving our own chances for survival.

The few instances in which man has looked to his fellow animals for ideas follow a discernible pattern that is promising. He has been able to improve the design of surface ships and submarines by studying live fishes swimming against the strong current in a river. He has gained an understanding of many important principles by observing the flight of birds, without having to construct airplanes out of bones, flesh and feathers. In each case he has devised substitutes that match his personal needs, by applying to his parallel inventions the natural laws discoverable from animal activities. He has realized that animals preceded him in solving problems of rapid movement in the realms of air and water. He can use many additional features fundamental to other abilities of animals. Nowhere is this transfer of discoveries more inviting than in extending man's own sensory world. It is far less costly to become an ingenious apprentice, watching how an animal survives, than to work out each problem separately.

A major breakthrough seems imminent in the field of communications. Already we have learned to interpret the dances of honeybees, to read bee-to-bee messages through a pane of red glass in the side of a hive. We know, too, that bee language has its dialects—like folk dances—and that they can introduce confusion if a well-traveled honeybee from southern Italy tries to impart information about the whereabouts of food to a stay-at-home in northern Germany. Similar provincialism is evident in America, in that a tree frog from Manitoba cannot compete successfully with a local vocalist of the same species for the attention of a female in a Georgia swamp. Nor do bird calls, recorded in one place, have a uniform meaning for birds of the identical kind in different parts of the country.

Interspecies communication, long a prerogative of the hunter, is now being extended to messages on a trial basis between man and honeybee. Success with porpoises too may be near, for these swimming mammals have been recognized as having a brain, vocal apparatus and hearing that may rival our own. In captivity they co-operate readily with one another and with man. Nowhere else, in fact, is there such a tempting opportunity to decipher a nonhuman approximation of speech as in porpoise calls under water. By finding features in common between the operation of a porpoise's brain and a man's, we stand a good chance of discovering the essential basis for elusive qualities such as memory, learning and intelligence.

Every new understanding of the nervous mechanisms in animals is likely to lead to fresh expansion of man's own sensory world. These achievements give us confidence that life for us is still open-ended, extremely variable, hemming us in on really few frontiers. By relying upon our own special heritage—our unique cerebral cortex and our relatively unspecialized bodies—we can benefit from personal experience begun at birth, as well as from the accumulated lore of civilization, and still further from the sensory riches of all other living animals. Through increasing our avenues of awareness we stand to gain these benefits, fortifying our faith in the future.

Something Extra

MUCH OF our own pleasure in thinking about the senses of animals and men comes through reading about discoveries, particularly when they correct old assumptions and uncover for us fresh avenues of awareness. It is impossible, of course, for any one person—or two—to read *all* the scientific reports bearing on this broad topic, or even to go thoughtfully and critically through all the pertinent books. But we suspect that some readers may wish to refer at first hand to some of the recent technical articles and books we have enjoyed. A partial listing follows, arranged by chapters in the book. Among them we have inserted a few references to more popular accounts, believing that these too may be helpful.

A SENSE OF WONDER

Sitwell, Dame Edith, 1958, "The Poet's Vision" in *Saturday Evening Post* 231 (20) : 29, 126-130 [Nov. 15, 1958] [reprinted in *Adventures of the Mind* (1960 : New York; Vintage Books, Inc.) pp. 117-129.]

CH. 1 THE "FIVE SENSES" AND A FEW MORE

Kanz, Ewald, 1951, "Neues über die Wetterwirkung auf die psycho-physische Reaktionslage des Menschen," in *Archiv f. physik. Therapie* 3 (4) : 211-215.

CH. 2   GUIDING TOUCHES

Barnes, H., 1955, "Further observations on rugophilic behaviour in *Balanus balanoides* (L.)," in *Vidensk. Meddel. Dansk naturhist. For. København* 117 : 341-348.

Buytendyk, F. J. J., 1953, "Toucher et être touché," in *Arch. Neerland. Zool.* 10, Suppl. 2 : 34-44.

Cooper, K. W., 1957, "Biology of eumenine wasps. V. Digital communication in wasps," in Jour. Exptl. Zool. 134 (3) : 469-513.

Digby, P. S. B., 1958, "Flight activity in the blowfly *Calliphora erythrocephala* in relation to wind speed, with special reference to adaptation" in *Jour. Exptl. Biol.* 35 (4) : 776-795.

Flanders, S. E., 1950, "Control of sex in the honeybee" in *Sci. Mo.* 71 (4) : 237-240.

Geldard, F. A., 1953, *The Human Senses* (New York: John Wiley & Sons).

Gohar, H. A. F., 1948, "Commensalism between fish and anemone" in *Publ. Marine Biol. Stat. Ghardaqua (Red Sea), Fouad I. Univ.,* 6 : 35-44.

Harlow, H. F., 1958, "The nature of love" in *Amer. Psychologist* 13 (12) : 673-685.

Harlow, H. F., 1959, "Love in infant monkeys" in *Sci. Amer.* 200 (6) : 67-74.

Harlow, H. F., and R. R. Zimmerman, 1959, "Affectional responses in the infant monkey" in *Science* 130 (3373) : 421-432.

Wilson, E. O., 1953, "The ecology of some North American decetine ants" in *Annals Ent. Soc. Amer.* 46 (4) : 479-495.

CH. 3   THE LANGUAGES OF VIBRATION

Blest, A. D., 1958, "Interaction between consecutive responses of a hemileucid moth, and the evolution of insect communication" in *Nature* 181 (4615) : 1077-1078.

Cosh, J. A., 1953, "Studies on the nature of vibration sense" in *Clin. Sci.* [London] 12 (2) : 131-151.

Frings, H., and F. Little, 1956, "Reactions of honey bees in the hive to simple sounds" in *Science* 125 (3238) : 122.

Geldard, F. A., 1960, "Some neglected possibilities of communication" in *Science* 131 (3413) : 1583-1588.

Jones, J. W., 1956, "The lateral line organs of fishes" in *Salmon and Trout Mag.* 147 : 166-169.

Lindauer, M., 1957, "Communication among the honeybees and stingless bees of India" in *Bee World* 38 (1) : 3-14; (2) : 34-39.

Prechtl, H. F. R., 1951, "Zur Paarungsbiologie einiger Molcharten" in *Ztschr. f. Tierpsychol.* 8 (3) : 337-347.

Saltpeter, M., and C. Walcott, 1958, "The anatomy of the vibration receptor of the spider" in *Anat. Rec.* 132 (3) : 501.

Schmieder, R. G., 1952, "Bees' dance directs the flight of the swarm" in *Ent. News* 63 (4) : 100-102.

Steche, Wolfgang, 1959, "How to talk to a bee" in *Time* for Feb. 9, p. 34.

Wolbarsht, M. L., and V. G. Dethier, 1958, "Electrical activity in chemoreceptors of the blowfly. I. Responses to chemical and mechanical stimulation" in *Jour. Gen. Physiol.* 42 : 393-412.

CH. 4   WHAT DO EARS TELL US?

van Békésy, G., 1957, "The ear" in *Sci. Amer.* 197 (2) : 66-78.

Bluemel, C. S., 1959, "Double-syllable words" in *Jour. Speech and Hearing Disorders* 24 (3) : 272-274.

Broadbent, D. E., 1960, "The sense of hearing" in *Nature* 188 (4747) : 268-270.

Deutsch, J. A., and J. K. Clarkson, 1959, "Nature of the vibrato and the control loop in singing" in *Nature* 183 (4655) : 167-168.

Frings, H., et al., 1958, "Reactions of American and French species of *Corvus* and *Larus* to recorded communication signals tested reciprocally" in *Ecology* 39 (1) : 126-131.

Frings, H., and M. Frings, 1959, "The language of crows" in *Sci. Amer.* 201 (5) : 119-131.

Jacobson, H., 1951, "Information and the human ear" in *Jour. Acoustical Soc. Amer.* 23 (4) : 463-471.

Miller, Loye, 1952, "Auditory recognition of predators" in *Condor* 54 (2) : 89-92.

Pierce, J. R., 1960, "Some work on hearing" in *Amer. Sci.* 48 (1) : 40-45.

Pierce, J. R., and E. E. David, Jr., 1958, *Man's World of Sound* (Garden City, N. Y.; Doubleday & Co.)

Pumphrey, R. J., 1950, "Upper limit of frequency for human hearing" in *Nature* 166 (4222) : 571.

Thomas, E. M., 1959, *The Harmless People* (New York: A. A. Knopf, Inc.)

CH. 5 THE NOISY WORLD OF THE SKIN DIVER

Dobrin, M. B., 1947, "Measurements of underwater noise produced by marine life" in *Science* 105 (2714) : 19-23.

Dobrin, M. B., 1949, "Recording sounds of undersea life" in *Trans. N. Y. Acad. Sci.* 11 (2) : 91-96.

Fish, M. P., 1956, "Animal sounds in the sea" in *Sci. Amer.* 194 (4) : 93-102.

Fish, M. P., A. S. Kelsey, Jr., and W. H. Mowbray, 1952, "Studies on the production of underwater sound by North Atlantic coastal fishes" in *Jour. Marine Res.* 11 (2) : 180-193.

Fish, M. P., and W. H. Mowbray, 1959, "The production of underwater sound by *Opsanus* sp., a new toadfish from Bimini, Bahamas" in *Zoologica* [New York] 44 (2) : 71-76.

Gray, G.-A., and H. Winn, 1958, "The sound production and behavior of the guarding male toadfish (*Opsanus tau*)" in *Anat. Rec.* 132 (3) : 446.

Kellogg, W. N., 1953, "Ultrasonic hearing in the porpoise, *Tursiops truncatus*" in *Jour. Comp. Physiol. & Psych.* 46 (6) : 446-450.

Kellogg, W. N., and R. Kohler, 1952, "Responses of the porpoise to ultrasonic frequencies" in *Science* 116 (3010) : 250-252.

Kleerekoper, H., and E. C. Chagnon, 1954, "Hearing in fish, with special reference to *Semotilus atromaculatus atromaculatus* (Mitchill)" in *Jour. Fish. Res. Bd. Canada* 11 (2) : 130-152.

Lilly, J. C., 1961, *Man and Dolphin* (Garden City, N.Y.; Doubleday & Co.)

Moulton, J. M., 1960, "Swimming sounds and the schooling of fishes" in *Biol. Bull.* 119 (2) : 210-223.

Rough, G. E., 1954, "The frequency range of mechanical vibrations perceived by three species of freshwater fish" in *Copeia* 1954 (3) : 191-194.

Schevill, W. E., and B. Lawrence, 1949, "Underwater listening to the white porpoise (*Delphinapterus leucas*)" in *Science* 109 (2824) : 143-144.

Schevill, W. E., and B. Lawrence, 1953, "High-frequency auditory response of a bottlenosed porpoise, *Tursiops truncatus* (Montagu) in *Jour. Acoustical Soc. Amer.* 25 (5) : 1016-1017.

Schevill, W. E., and B. Lawrence, 1953, "Auditory response of a bottlenosed porpoise, *Tursiops truncatus*, to frequencies above 100 kc." in *Jour. Exptl. Zool.* 124 (1) : 147-165.

Stout, J. and H. E. W. Winn, 1958, "The reproductive behavior and sound production of the satinfin shiner" in *Anat. Rec.* 132 (3) : 511.

Tavolga, W. N., 1958, "Significance of underwater sounds produced by males of the gobiid fish, *Bathygobius soporator*" in *Physiol. Zool.* 31 (4) : 259-271.

Tavolga, W. N., 1960, "Foghorn sounds beneath the sea" in *Natural History* [New York] 69 (3) : 44-51.

Wood, F. G., 1953, "Underwater sound production and concurrent behavior of captive porpoises, *Tursiops truncatus* and *Stenella plagiodon*" in *Bull. Marine Sci. Gulf & Caribb.* 3 (2) : 120-133.

CH. 6   THE SOUNDS OF THE SEASONS

Alexander, A. J., 1958, "On the stridulation of scorpions" in *Behaviour* 12 (4) : 339-352.

Alexander, R. D., 1957, "The song relationships of four species of ground crickets (Orthoptera: Gryllidae: *Nemobius*)" in *Ohio Jour. Sci.* 57 (3) : 153-163.

Alexander, R. D., and T. E. Moore, 1958, "Studies on the acoustical behavior of seventeen-year cicadas (Homoptera: Cicadidae: *Magicicada*)" in *Ohio Jour. Sci.* 58 (2) : 107-127.

Blair, W. F., 1958, "Mating call in the speciation of anuran amphibians" in *Amer. Nat.* 92 (862) : 27-51.

Borror, D. J., and C. R. Reese, 1956, "Vocal gymnastics in wood thrush songs" in *Ohio Jour. Sci.* 56 (3) : 177-182.

Busnel, R.-G. and B. DuMortier, 1955, "Etude du cycle génital du mâle d'*Ephippiger* et son rapport avec le comportement acoustique" in *Bull. Soc. Zool. France* 80 (1) : 23-26.

Eibl-Eibesfeldt, I., 1952, "Vergleichende Verhaltensstudien an Anuren. 1. Zur Paarungsbiologie des Laubfrosches, *Hyla arborea* L." in *Ztschr. f. Tierpsychol.* 9 (3) : 383-395.

Frings, H., and M. Frings, 1956, "Reactions to sounds by the wood nymph butterfly, *Cercyonis pegala*" in *Annals Entom. Soc. Amer.* 49 (6) : 611-617.

Gaul, A.T., 1952, "Audio mimicry: an adjunct to color mimicry" in *Psyche* 59 (2) : 82-83.

Haskell, P. T., 1957, "The influence of flight noise on behavior in the desert locust *Schistocerca gregaria* (Forsk.)" in *Jour. Insect Physiol.* 1 (1) : 52-75.

Kilham, L., 1959, "Mutual tapping of the red-headed woodpecker" in *Auk* 76 (2) : 235-236.

Kleerekoper, H., and K. Sibabin, 1959, "Hearing in frogs (*Rana pipiens* and *R. clamitans*)" in *Ztschr. f. vergl. Physiol.* 41 (4) : 490-499.

Neff, W. D., and J. E. Hind, 1955, "Auditory thresholds of the cat" in *Jour. Acoustical Soc. Amer.* 27 (3) : 480-483.

Neill, W. T., 1958, "The varied calls of the barking treefrog, *Hyla gratiosa* LeConte" in *Copeia* 1958 (1) : 44-46.

Perdeck, A. C., 1951, [Experiments with short-horned grasshoppers] in *Levende Natuur* 54 (9) : 165-172.

Pierce, G. W., 1948, *The Songs of Insects* (Cambridge, Mass.: Harvard Univ. Press).

Pringle, J. W. S., 1956, "Insect song" in *Endeavour* 15 (58) : 68-72.

Thorpe, W. H., 1956, "The language of birds" in *Sci. Amer.* 195 (4) : 128-138.

Wishart, G., and D. F. Riordan, 1959, "Flight responses to various sounds by adult males of *Aedes aegypti* (L.) (Diptera: Culicidae)" *Canadian Entom.* 91 (3) : 181-191.

Woods, E. F., 1959, "Electronic prediction of swarming in bees" in *Nature* 184 (4690) : 842:844.

CH. 7   ECHOES OF IMPORTANCE

Backus, R. H., 1959, "Echo ranging in the porpoise" in *Science* 129 (3350) : 730. And reply, same page, by W. N. Kellogg.

Bloedel, P., 1955, "Hunting methods of fish-eating bats, particularly *Noctilio leporinus*" in *Jour. Mammal.* 36 (3) : 390-399.

Fraser, F. C., and P. E. Purves, 1954, "Hearing in cetaceans" in *Bull. Brit. Mus. (Nat. Hist.), Zool.* 2 (5) : 1010-114.

Fraser, F. C., and P. E. Purves, 1959, "Hearing in whales" in *Endeavour* 18 (70) : 93-98.

Frings, H., and M. Frings, 1957, "Duplex nature of reception of simple sounds in the scape moth, *Ctenucha virginica*" in *Science* 126 (3262) : 24.

Gould, E., 1955, "The feeding efficiency of insectivorous bats" in *Jour. Mammal.* 36 (3) : 399-407.

Griffin, D. R., 1951, "Audible and ultrasonic sounds of bats" in *Experientia* 7 (12) : 448-453.

Griffin, D. R., 1955, "Hearing and acoustic orientation in marine animals" in *Deep-Sea Res.* 3 (Suppl) : 406-417.

Griffin, D. R., 1958, *Listening in the Dark; the Acoustic Orientation of Bats and Men* (New Haven: Yale Univ. Press).

Griffin, D. R., 1959, *Echoes of Bats and Men* (Garden City, N.Y.: Doubleday & Co.).

Grinnell, A. D., and D. R. Griffin, 1958, "The sensitivity of echolocation in bats" in *Biol. Bull.* 114 (1) : 10-22.

van Heel, W. H. D., 1959, "Audio-direction finding in the porpoise (*Phocaena phocaena*)" in *Nature* 183 (4667) : 1063.

Kahmann, N., and K. Ostermann, 1951, "Wahrnehmen und Hervorbringen hoher Töne bei kleinen Säugetieren" in *Experientia* 7 (7) : 268-269.

Kellogg, W. N., 1958, "Echo ranging in the porpoise" in *Science* 128 (3330) : 982-988.

Kellogg, W. N., 1959, "Auditory perception of submerged objects by porpoises" in *Jour. Acoustical Soc. Amer.* 31 (1) : 1-5.

Kellogg, W. N., 1961, *Porpoises and Sonar* (Chicago: Univ. of Chicago Press).

Kellogg, W. N., and R. Kohler, "Reactions of the porpoise to ultrasonic frequencies" in *Science* 116 (3010) : 250-252.

Kellogg, W. N., R. Kohler, and H. N. Morris, 1953, "Porpoise sounds as sonar signals" in *Science* 117 (3036) : 239-243.

Marler, P., 1955, "Characteristics of some animal calls" in *Nature* 176 (4470) : 6-8.

Medway, Lord, 1959 "Echo-location among *Collocalia*" in *Nature* 184

286 THE SENSES OF ANIMALS AND MEN

(4696) : 1352-1353.

Norris, K. S., et al., 1961, "An experimental demonstration of echo-locating behavior in the porpoise, *Tursiops truncatus* (Montagu)" in *Biol. Bull.* 120 (2) : 163-176.

Novick, A., 1958, "Orientation in paleotropical bats. I. Microchiroptera" in *Jour. Exptl. Zool.* 138 (1) : 81-153.

Novick, A., 1958, "Orientation in paleotropical bats. II. Megachiroptera" in *Jour. Exptl. Zool.* 137 (3) : 443-462.

Novick, A., 1959, "Acoustic orientation in the swiftlet" in *Biol. Bull.* 117 (3) : 497-503.

Pye, J. D., 1961, "Echolocation by bats" in *Endeavour* 20 (78) : 101-111.

Riley, D. A., and M. R. Rosenzweig, 1957, "Echo-location in rats" in *Jour. Comp. & Physiol. Psychol.* 50 : 323-328.

Roeder, K. D., and A. E. Treat, 1957, "Ultrasonic reception by the tympanic organ of noctuid moths" in *Jour. Exptl. Zool.* 134 (1) : 127-158.

Sandel, T. T., et al., 1955, "Localization of sound from single and paired sources" in *Jour. Acoustical Soc. Amer.* 27 (5) : 842-852.

Schevill, W. E., and A. F. McBride, 1956, "Evidence for echolocation by cetaceans" in *Deep-Sea Res.* 3 (2) 153-154.

Schevill, W. E., and B. Lawrence, 1956, "Food-finding by a captive porpoise (*Tursiops truncatus*)" in *Breviora Mus. Comp. Zöol.* [Harvard Univ.] 53 : 1-15.

Treat, A. E., 1955, "The response to sound in certain Lepidoptera" in *Annals Entom. Soc. Amer.* 48 (4) : 272-284.

Vogelberg, L., and F. Krüger, 1951, "Versuche über die Richtungsorientierung bei weissen Mäusen and Ratten" in *Ztschr. f. Tierpsychol.* 8 (2) : 293-321.

CH. 8   HOT OR COLD?

Adler, S., 1959, "Darwin's illness" in *Nature* 184 (4693) : 1102-1103.

Andrews, E. A., 1955, "Some work of the periodical cicada" in *Jour. Washington Acad. Sci.* 45 (1) : 20-29.

Benzinger, T. H., 1961, "The human thermostat" in *Sci. Amer.* 204 (1) : 134-147.

Bullock, T. H., and F. P. J. Diecke, 1956, "Properties of an infra-red receptor" in *Jour. Physiol.* 134 (1) : 47-87.

Hock, R. J., and B. G. Covino, 1958, "Hypothermia" in *Sci. Amer.* 198 (3) : 104-114.

Kuhn, R. A., 1961, "Low-temperature surgery" in *Family Circle* (May 1961) : 25, 74, 76, 110.

Rozin, P. N., and Jean Mayer, 1961, "Thermal reinforcement and thermoregulatory behavior in goldfish, *Carassius auratus*" in *Science* 134 (3483) : 942-943.

Simpson, J., 1961, "Nest climate regulation in honey bee colonies" in *Science* 133 (3461) : 1327-1333.

Weiss, B., and V. G. Laties, 1961, "Behavioral thermoregulation" in *Science* 133 (3461) : 1338-1344.

CH. 9   SHOCKING INFORMATION

Grundfest, H., 1960, "Electric fishes" in *Sci. Amer.* 203 (4) : 115-124.

Keynes, R. D., 1956, "The generation of electricity by fishes" in *Endeavour* 15 (57) : 215-222.

Kleerekoper, H., 1958, "The localization of prey by the sea lamprey, *Petromyzon marinus* (L.)" in *Anat. Rec.* 132 (3) : 464.

Lissmann, H. W., 1958, "On the function and evolution of electric organs in fish" in *Jour. Exptl. Biol.* 35 (1) : 156-191.

Lissmann, H. W., and K. E. Machin, 1958, "The mechanism of object location in *Gymnarchus niloticus* and similar fish" in *Jour. Exptl. Biol.* 35 (2) : 451-486.

Wright, P. G., 1958, "An electrical receptor in fishes" in *Nature* 181 (4601) : 64-65.

CH. 10   THE IMPORTANCE OF ODORS

Bang, B. G., 1960, "Anatomical evidence for olfactory function in some species of birds" in *Nature* 188 (4750) : 547-549.

Bardach, J. E., H. E. Winn, and D. W. Menzel, 1959, "The role of the senses in the feeding of the nocturnal reef predators *Gymnothorax moringa* and *G. vicinus*" in *Copeia* 1959 (2) : 133-139.

Beach, F. A., and J. Jaynes, 1956, "Studies of maternal retrieving in rats. I. Recognition of young" in *Jour. Mammal.* 37 (2) : 177-180.

Bedichek, Roy, 1960, *The Sense of Smell* (Garden City, N. Y.: Doubleday & Co.)

Bruce, H. M., and D. M. V. Parrott, 1960, "Role of olfactory sense in pregnancy block by strange males" in *Science* 131 (3412) : 1526.

Butler, C. G., 1954, "The method and importance of the recognition by a colony of honeybees (*A. mellifera*) of the presence of its queen" in *Trans. Roy. Entom. Soc. London* 105 (2) : 11-29.

Carthy, J. D., 1958, *An Introduction to the Behaviour of Invertebrates* (London: George Allen & Unwin, Ltd.)

Chin, Chun-Ten, 1950, "Studies on the physiological relations between the larvae of *Leptinotarsa decimlineata* Say and some solanaceous plants" (Wageningen, Netherlands: H. Veeman & Zonen)

Deinse, J. B. v., L. B. W. Jongkees, and J. Klijn, 1954, "Olfactory nystagmus of the head" in *Acta Oto-laryngol.* 44 (3) : 233-236.

Dethier, V. G., 1954, "The physiology of olfaction in insects" in *Annals N. Y. Acad. Sci.* 58 (2) : 139-155.

El-Baradi, A. F., and G. H. Bourne, 1951, "Localization of gustatory and olfactory enzymes in the rabbit, and the problems of taste and smell" in *Nature* 168 (4284) : 977-979.

Goetzl, F. R., M. S. Abel, and A. J. Ahokas, 1950, "Occurrence in normal individuals of diurnal variations in olfactory acuity" in *Jour. Appl. Physiol.* 2 (10) : 553-562.

Hasler, A. D., 1954, "Odour perception and orientation in fishes" in *Jour. Fisheries Res. Bd. Canada* 11 (2) : 107-129.

Jacobson, M., M. Beroza, and W. A. Jones, 1960, "Isolation, identification and synthesis of the sex attractant of gypsy moth" in *Science* 132 (3433) : 1011.

Kalmus, H., 1955, "The discrimination by the nose of the dog of individual human odours and in particular the odours of twins" in *Brit. Jour. Animal Behaviour* 3 (1) : 25-31.

Köhler, F., 1955, "Wache und Volksduft im Bienenstaat" in *Ztschr. f. Bienenforsch.* 3 (3) : 57-63.

LeMagnen, J., 1952, "Les phénomenes olfacto-sexuels chez l'homme" in *Arch. Sci. Physiol.* 6 (2) : 125-160.

LeMagnen, J., 1952, "Les phénomenes olfacto-sexuels chez le rat blanc" in *Arch. Sci. Physiol.* 6 (4) : 295-331.

Spillane, A. E., 1954, "Feeding habits of the orchard spider" in *Victorian Nat.* 71 (3) : 50.

Whitten, W. K., 1956, "Modification of the mouse oestrous cycle by external stimuli associated with the male" in *Jour. Endocrinol.* 13 (4) : 399-404.

CH. 11   THE LIMITS OF TASTE

Bullock, T. H., 1953, "Predator recognition and escape responses of some intertidal gastropods in presence of starfish" in *Behaviour* 5 (2) : 1-11.

Carthy, J. D., 1958, *An Introduction to the Behaviour of Invertebrates* (London: George Allen & Unwin, Ltd.)

Deutsch, J. A., and A. D. Jones, 1959, "The water-salt receptor and preference in the rat" in *Nature* 183 (4673) : 1472.

Frings, H., 1951, "Sweet taste in the cat and the taste-spectrum" in *Experientia* 7 (11) : 424-426.

Geldard, F. A., 1953, *The Human Senses* (New York: John Wiley & Sons).

Kalmus, H., 1958, "The chemical senses" in *Sci. Amer.* 198 (4) : 97-106.

Karlson, P., and M. Lüscher, 1959, " 'Pheromones': A new term for a class of biologically active substances" in *Nature* 183 (4653) : 55-56.

Miles, P. W., 1958, "Contact chemoreception in some Heteroptera, including chemoreception internal to the stylet food canal" in *Jour. Insect Physiol.* 2 (4) : 338-347.

Pfaffman, C., 1959, "The sense of taste" as Chapter XX (pp. 507-533) in *Handbook of Physiology*, Section 1. Neurophysiology, vol. 1 (Washington, D.C.: Amer. Physiol. Soc.)

Roth, L. M., and E. R. Willis, 1952, "A study of cockroach behavior" in *Amer. Midland Nat.* 47 (1) : 66-129.

van Tyne, J., and A. J. Berger, 1959, *Fundamentals of Ornithology* (New York: John Wiley & Sons), pp. 114, 257-259.

Zayko, N. S., 1956, [Regular phenomena of the functional activity of the human gustatory receptor apparatus] in *Biull. Eksp. Biol. i. Met.* 41 (1) : 19-22.

Zotterman, Y., and H. Diamant, 1959, "Has water a specific taste?" in *Nature* 183 (4655) : 191-192.

CH. 12   THE MYSTERY OF THIRST

Brown, Harrison, 1954, *The Challenge of Man's Future* (New York: Viking Press) pp. 168-172.

Lindauer, M., 1955, "The water economy and temperature regulation of the honeybee colony" in *Bee World* 36 (4) : 62-72; (5) : 81-92; (6) : 105-111.

Rainey, R. C., 1951, "Weather and the movements of locust swarms: a new hypothesis" in *Nature* 168 (4286) : 1057-1060.

Schmidt-Nielsen, K., 1959, "The physiology of the camel" in *Sci. Amer.* 201 (6) : 140-151.

Smith, H. W., 1953, *From Fish to Philosopher* (Boston: Little, Brown & Co.)

Stellar, E., R. Hyman, and S. Samet, 1954, "Gastric factors controlling water- and salt-solution-drinking" in *Jour. Comp. & Physiol. Psychol.* 47 (3) : 220-226.

Wolf, A. V., "Thirst" in *Sci. Amer.* 194 (1) : 70-76.

Wolf, A. V., 1958, *Thirst* (Springfield, Ill.: C. C. Thomas).

Zotterman, Y., 1950, "The water taste of the frog" in *Experientia* 6 (2) : 57-58.

CH. 13   OBSCURE SENSES

Ardö, P., 1958, "On the feeding habits of the Scandinavian mosquitoes" in *Opuscula Entom.* 23 (3) : 171-191.

Armstrong, E. A., 1954, "The behavior of birds in continuous daylight" in *Ibis* 96 (1) : 1-30.

Balch, C. C., 1955, "Sleep in ruminants" in *Nature* 175 (4465) : 940-941.

Friedmann, H., 1955, "The honey-guides" in *Bull. U. S. Nat. Mus.* 208 : 1-192.

Friedmann, H., 1958, "Cerophagy in the honey-guides and its microbiological implications" in *Anat. Rec.* 132 (3) : 440.

Hess, E. H., and J. M. Polt, 1960, "Pupil size as related to interest value of visual stimuli" in *Science* 132 (3423) : 349-350.

Kleitman, N., 1960, "Patterns of dreaming" in *Sci. Amer.* 203 (5) : 82-88.

Lockley, R. M., 1960, "Social structure and stress in the rabbit warren" in *The New Scientist* (Dec. 15) : 1580-1583.

Newkirk, M. R., 1957, "On the black-topped hangingfly (Mecoptera, Bittacidae)" in *Annals Entom. Soc. Amer.* 50 (3) : 302-306.

Olds, J., 1956, "Pleasure centers in the brain" in *Sci. Amer.* 195 (4) : 105-116.

Qazim, S. Z., 1955, "Rearing experiments on marine teleost larvae and evidence of their need for sleep" in *Nature* 175 (4448) : 217-218.

Schremmer, F., 1955, "Beobachtungen über die Nachtruhe bei Hymenopteren, insbesondere die Männschenschlafgesellschaften von *Halictus*" in *Österreich. zool. Ztschr.* 6 (½) : 70-89.

CH. 14   WHAT TIME IS IT?

Brown, F. A. Jr., M. Webb, and M. F. Bennett, 1955, "Proof for an endogenous component in persistent solar and lunar rhythmicity in organisms" in *Proc. Nat. Acad. Sci.* 41 (2) : 92-100.

Cloudsley-Thompson, J. L., 1953, "Studies in diurnal rhythms. III. Photoperiodism in the cockroach *Periplaneta americana* (L.)" in *Ann. & Mag. Nat. Hist.* 6 (69) : 705-712.

Cloudsley-Thompson, J. L., 1959, "Animal clocks" in *Nature* 184 (4689) : 763-765.

Hauenschild, C., 1955, "Photoperiodizität als Ursache des von der Mondphase abhängigen Metamorphose-Rhythmus bei dem Polychaeten *Platynereis dumerlii*" in *Ztschr. f. Naturforsch.* 10b (11) : 658-662.

Mattingly, P. F., 1952, "Recent work on cyclical behaviour in the Nematocera" in *Trans. IXth Internat. Congr. Entom.* 1 : 375-378.

Pittendrigh, C. S., 1954, "On temperature independence in the clock system controlling emergence time in *Drosophila*" in *Proc. Nat. Acad. Sci.* 40 : 1018-1029.

Roberts, S. K. de F., 1956, " 'Clock' controlled activity rhythms in the fruit fly" in *Science* 124 (3213) : 172.

Roberts, S. K. de F., 1958, "The cockroach clock—effects of light and temperature" in *Anat. Rec.* 132 (3) : 494.

Schremmer, F., 1955, "Beobachtungen über die Nachtruhe bei Hymenopteren, insbesondere die Männschenschlafgesellschaften von *Halictus*" in *Österreich. zool. Ztschr.* 6 (½) : 70-89.

Turner, H. J. Jr., and D. L. Belding, 1957, "The tidal migrations of *Donax variabilis* Say" in *Limnol. and Oceanography* 1 (2) : 120-124.

CH. 15   HABITUAL MOVEMENTS

Aronson, L. R., 1951, "Orientation and jumping behavior in the gobiid fish, *Bathygobius soporator*" in *Amer. Mus. Novitates* 1486 : 1-21.

Geldard, F. A., 1953, *The Human Senses* (New York: John Wiley & Sons).

Gerard, R. W., 1953, "What is memory?" in *Sci. Amer.* 189 (3) : 118-126.

Griffin, D. R., 1958, *Listening in the Dark: the Acoustic Orientation of Bats and Men* (New Haven: Yale Univ. Press).

Klosovsky, B. N., and E. N. Kosmarskaya, 1955, [Behavior of animals after complete elimination of visual, auditory, olfactory and vestibular receptors at an early age] in *Biull. Eksptl. Biol. i. Med.* 39 (9) : 3-6.

Rose, J. E., and V. B. Mountcastle, 1959, "Touch and kinesis" as Chapter XVII (pp. 387-429) in *Handbook of Physiology*, Section 1, Neurophysiology, vol. 1 (Washington, D.C.: Amer. Physiol. Soc.)

CH. 16   WHICH SIDE IS UP?

Autrum, H., 1959, "Nonphotic receptors in lower forms" as Chapter XVI (pp. 369-385) in *Handbook of Physiology*, Section 1, Neurophysiology, vol. 1 (Washington, D.C.: Amer. Physiol. Soc.)

Boycott, B. B., and J. Z. Young, 1956, "Reactions to shape in *Octopus vulgaris*" in *Proc. Zool. Soc. London* 126 : 491-547.

Cohen, M. J., 1955, "The function of receptors in the statocyst of the lobster *Homarus americanus*" in *Jour. Physiol.* 130 (1) : 9-34.

Dijkgraaf, S., 1952, "Bau und Funktionen der Seitenorgane und des

Ohrlabyrinths bei Fischen" in *Experientia* 8 (6) : 205-216.

Mittelstädt, H., 1950, "Physiologie des Gleichgewichtssinnes bei fliegenden Libellen," in *Ztschr. f. vergl. Physiol.* 32 : 422-463.

Rabe, W., 1953, "Beiträge zum Orientierungsproblem des Wasserwanzen" in *Ztschr. f. allg. Physiol.* 20 : 1-34.

Schneider, G., 1958, "Static sense of *Calliphora* and the physical stabilizing effect of the halteres" in *Nature* 181 (4619) : 1355-1356.

Schöne, H., 1951, "Die statische Gleichgewichtsorientierung dekapoder Crustacean" in *Verhand. deutsch. Ges. Wilhelmshaven* 1951 : 157-162.

Wit, G. de, 1953, "Sea sickness (motion sickness). A labyrinthological study" in *Acta Oto-laryngol.* (Suppl.) 108 : 7-55.

CH. 17   WHICH WAY TO TURN?

Bainbridge, R., and T. H. Waterman, 1958, "Turbidity and the polarized light orientation of the crustacean *Mysidium*" in *Jour. Exptl. Biol.* 35 (3) : 487-493.

Brown, F. A. Jr., et al., 1960, "Magnetic response of an organism and its solar relationships" in *Biol. Bull.* 118 (3) : 367-392.

Brown, F. A. Jr., et al., 1960, "A magnetic compass response of an organism" in *Biol. Bull.* 119 (1) : 65-74.

Burdon-Jones, C., and G. H. Charles, 1958, "Light reactions of littoral gastropods" in *Nature* 181 (4602) : 129-131.

Carthy, J. D., 1957, "Polarised light and animals" in *Discovery* 18 (3) : 105-109.

Carthy, J. D., 1958, *An Introduction to the Behaviour of Invertebrates* (London: George Allen & Unwin Ltd.)

Enright, J. T., 1961, "Lunar orientation of *Orchestoidea corniculata* Stout (Amphipoda)" in *Biol. Bull.* 120 (2) : 148-156.

von Frisch, K., 1960, *Bees: Their Vision, Chemical Senses and Language* (Ithaca, N.Y.: Cornell Univ. Press).

Griffin, D. R., 1953, "Sensory physiology and the orientation of animals" in *Amer. Scientist* 41 (2) : 209-244.

Hasler, A. D., 1956, "Perception of pathways by fishes in migration" in *Quart. Rev. Biol.* 31 (3) : 200-209.

Hasler, A. D., et al., 1958, "Sun-orientation and homing in fishes" in *Limnol. and Oceanogr.* 3 (4) : 353-361.

Kalmus, H., 1957, "The sun navigation of bees in the southern hemisphere" in *Bee World* 38 (2) : 29-33.

Kalmus, H., 1959, "Orientation of animals to polarized light" in *Nature* 184 (4682) : 228-230.

Kowalski, K., and R. J. Wojtusiak, 1952, "Homing experiments on bats. I" in *Bull. Internat. Acad. Polonaise Sci. et Lettres* Ser. B 2, Zool. 1951 (1/2) : 33-56.

Medioni, J., 1956, "L'orientation 'astronomique' des arthropodes et des oiseaux" in *Ann. Biol.* 32 (1/2) : 37-67.

Milne, L. J., and M. Milne, 1958, *Paths Across the Earth* (New York: Harper & Bros.)

Moody, M. F., and J. R. Parriss, 1960, "Discrimination of polarized light by *Octopus*" in *Nature* 186 (4726) : 839-840.

Mueller, H. C., and J. T. Emlen Jr., 1957, "Homing in bats" in *Science* 126 (3268) : 307-308.

Sauer, F., 1957, "Die Sternenorientierung nächtlich ziehender Grasmücken (*Sylvia atricapilla*, Borin und Curruca)" in *Ztschr. f. Tierpsychol.* 14 (1) : 29-70.

Schmidt-Koenig, K., 1960, "The sun azimuth compass: one factor in the orientation of homing pigeons" in *Science* 131 (3403) : 826-828.

Stephens, G. C., M. Fingerman, and F. A. Brown Jr., 1953, "The orientation of *Drosophila* to plane polarized light" in *Annals Entom. Soc. Amer.* 46 (1) : 75-83.

Twitty, V. C., 1959, "Migration and speciation in newts" in *Science* 130 (3391) : 1735-1743.

Williamson, D. O., 1951, "Studies in the biology of Talitridae (Crustacea, Amphipoda): Visual orientation in *Talitrus saltator*" in *Jour. Marine Biol. Assoc. U. K.* 30 (1) : 91-99.

CH. 18   VISION BY DAY

Allen, F., 1951, "The visual apparatus as an optical instrument" in *Sci. Mo.* 72 (2) : 71-74.

Alley, R., and H. Boyd, 1950, "Parent-young recognition in the coot" in *Ibis* 92 (1) : 46-51.

Campbell, F. W., 1954, "The minimum quantity of light required to elicit the accommodation reflex in man" in *Jour. Physiol.* 123 (2) : 357-366.

Davis, M., 1950, "Model planes and purple martins, *Progne subis*" in *Auk* 67 (4) : 518.

Ditchburn, R. W., D. H. Fender, and S. Mayne, 1959, "Vision with controlled movements of the retinal image" in *Jour. Physiol.* 145 : 98-107.

Donner, K. O., 1951, "The visual acuity of some passerine birds" in *Acta Zool. Fennica* 66 : 1-40.

Duke-Elder, Sir S., 1958, *The Eye in Evolution* (London: Henry Kimpton)

Eibl-Eibesfeldt, I., 1952, "Nahrungserwerb und Beutescheme der Erdkröte (*Bufo bufo* L.)" in *Behaviour* 4 (1) : 1-35.

Eltringham, H., 1923, *Butterfly Lore* (Oxford: Clarendon Press) pp. 126-128.

Frings, H., et al., 1955, "Auditory and visual mechanisms in food-finding behavior of the herring gull" in *Wilson Bull.* 67 (3) : 155-170.

Guhl, A. M., and L. L. Ortman, 1953, "Visual patterns in the recognition of individuals among chickens" in *Condor* 55 (6) : 287-298.

Kaess, W., and F. Kaess, 1960, "Perception of apparent motion in the common toad" in *Science* 132 (3422) : 953.

Koenig, L., 1951, "Beiträge zu einem Aktionssystem des Bienenfressers (*Merops apiaster* L.)" in *Ztschr. f. Tierpsychol.* 8 (2) : 169-210.

Portmann, A., 1959, *Animal Camouflage* (Ann Arbor, Mich.: Univ. Michigan Press).

Smith, W. M., J. W. McCrary, and K. U. Smith, 1960, "Delayed visual feedback and behavior" in *Science* 132 (3433) : 1013-1014.

Sperry, R. W., 1956, "The eye and the brain" in *Sci. Amer.* 194 (5) : 48-52.

Wald, G., 1950, "Eye and camera" in *Sci. Amer.* 183 (2) : 32-41.

Walls, G., 1942, *The Vertebrate Eye* (Bloomfield Hills, Mich.: Cranbrook Inst. Sci.).

CH. 19   SEEING AT NIGHT

Duke-Elder, Sir S., 1958, *The Eye in Evolution* (London: Henry Kimpton).

Leibowitz, H., and T. Hartman, 1959, "Magnitude of the moon illusion as a function of the age of the observer" in *Science* 130 (3375) : 569-570.

Milne, L. J., and M. Milne, 1956, *The World of Night* (New York: Harper & Bros.).

Walls, G., 1942, *The Vertebrate Eye* (Bloomfield Hills, Mich.: Cranbrook Inst. Sci.).

Weale, R. A., 1955, "The absolute threshold of vision" in *Physiol. Rev.* 35 (1) : 233-246.

CH. 20   ANIMALS WITH FLASHLAMPS

Clarke, G. L., and R. H. Backus, 1956, "Measurements of light penetration in relation to vertical migration and records of luminescence of deep-sea animals" in *Deep-Sea Res.* 4 (1) : 1-14.

Colman, J. S., 1960, "A possible function of planktonic photophores" in *Nature* 185 (4706) : 112.

Denton, E. J., and F. J. Warren, 1957, "The photosensitive pigments in the retinae of deep-sea fish" in *Jour Marine Biol. Assoc. U. K.* 36 (3) : 651-662.

Duke-Elder, Sir S., 1958, *The Eye in Evolution* (London: Henry Kimpton).

Günther, K., and K. Deckert, 1956, *Creatures of the Deep Sea* [translated by E. W. Dickes] (London: George Allen & Unwin, Ltd.).

Harvey, E. N., 1952, *Bioluminescence* (New York: Academic Press, Inc.).

Harvey, E. N., 1957, "The luminous organs of fishes" as Chapt. VI (pp. 345-366) in *The Physiology of Fishes*, M. Brown edit. (New York: Academic Press, Inc.), vol. 2.

Kampa, E., and B. P. Boden, 1957, "Light generation in a sonic-scattering layer" in *Deep-Sea Res.* 4 (2) : 73-92.

Marshall, N. B., 1954, *Aspects of Deep Sea Biology* (New York: Philosophical Library, Inc.).

Nicol, J. A. C., 1958, "Luminescence in *Noctiluca*" in *Jour. Marine Biol. Assoc. U. K.* 37 (2) : 535-549.

Nicol, J. A. C., 1958, "Observations on luminescence in pelagic animals" in *Jour. Marine Biol. Assoc. U. K.* 37 (3) : 705-752.

Wald, G., P. K. Brown, and P. S. Brown, "Visual pigments and depth of habitat of marine fishes" in *Nature* 180 (4593) : 969-971.

Zenkevich, L. A., and J. A. Birstein, 1956, "Studies of the deep water fauna and related problems" in *Deep-Sea Res.* 4 (1) : 54-64.

CH. 21   SURVIVAL

DuBrul, E. L., 1958, "Brain and behavior" in *Anat. Rec.* 132 (3) : 428.

Holzman, B. G., 1960, "Birds, bees and ballistic beasts" in *Science* 132 (3430) : 793-794.

Milne, L. J., and M. Milne, 1960, *The Balance of Nature* (New York: A. Knopf, Inc.).

Urquhart, F. A., 1960, *The Monarch Butterfly* (Toronto, Canada: Univ. Toronto Press).

Index

Lorus *and* Margery Milne

LORUS and MARGERY MILNE, professors and exploring scientists, have worked together since their college days. They have lectured at a number of universities, including the Scripps Institution of Oceanography; have been visiting lecturers in South Africa on the United States-South Africa Leader Exchange Program; and have lectured for the National Audubon Society. For their work they have received a science-writing award from the American Association for the Advancement of Science, a Nash Conservation Award, a Saxton Literary Fellowship, and a Faculty Fellowship from the Fund for Advancement of Education. Their travels have taken them over 300,000 miles through four continents. Photographs they have made have appeared in many newspapers and magazines here and abroad. Their articles have been published in *The American Scholar*, *Atlantic Monthly*, *Audubon Magazine*, *Natural History*, *Scientific American* and other national periodicals. Among their twelve books, the most recent are *Paths Across the Earth*, 1958. *Animal Life* and *Plant Life*, both published in 1959, *The Balance of Nature*, 1960, *The Lower Animals: Living Invertebrates of the World*, 1960 and *The Mountains*, 1962. Lorus J. Milne was born in Toronto, Canada, and is now a citizen of the United States. He attended the University of Toronto, where he was named a Gold Medalist for his work in biology and received his Ph.D. from Harvard University. Margery Milne, a native of New York City, attended Columbia University and received her M.A. and Ph.D. from Radcliffe College. Mr. and Mrs. Milne live in Durham, New Hampshire.